SUSTAINING THE DRIVE TO OVERCOME THE GLOBAL IMPACT OF NEGLECTED TROPICAL DISEASES

SECOND WHO REPORT ON NEGLECTED TROPICAL DISEASES

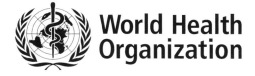
World Health Organization

WHO Library Cataloguing-in-Publication Data

Sustaining the drive to overcome the global impact of neglected tropical diseases: second WHO report on neglected diseases.

1 Tropical medicine - trends. 2.Neglected diseases. 3.Poverty areas. 4.Parasitic diseases. 5.Developing countries. 6.Annual reports. I.World Health Organization.

ISBN 978 92 4 156454 0   (NLM classification: WC 680)

Sustaining the drive to overcome the global impact of neglected tropical diseases: second WHO report on neglected tropical diseases was produced under the overall direction and supervision of Dr Lorenzo Savioli (Director) and Dr Denis Daumerie (Programme Manager), WHO Department of Control of Neglected Tropical Diseases, with contributions from staff serving in the department.

Regional directors and members of their staff provided support and advice.

Valuable input in the form of contributions, peer review and suggestions were received from members of WHO's Strategic and Technical Advisory Group for Neglected Tropical Diseases.

The report was edited by Professor David WT Crompton.

Design, layout and figures: Patrick Tissot (WHO/NTD); maps by Alexei Mikhailov (WHO/NTD).
Cover: Patrick Tissot (WHO/NTD); adapted from an original idea by Denis Meissner (WHO/GRA).

Printed in France
WHO/HTM/NTD/2013.1

CONTENTS

HIGHLIGHTS

Sustaining the drive to overcome the global impact of neglected tropical diseases • Second WHO report on neglected tropical diseases

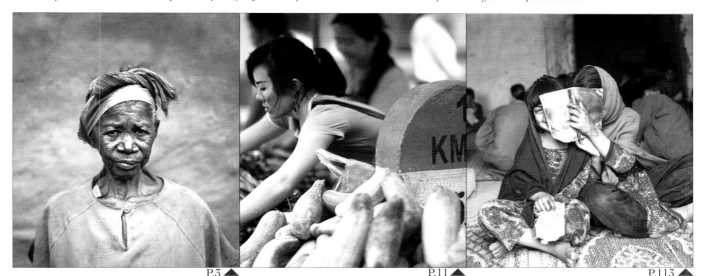

P.3 ▲   P.11 ▲   P.113 ▲

CONTENTS

CONTENTS

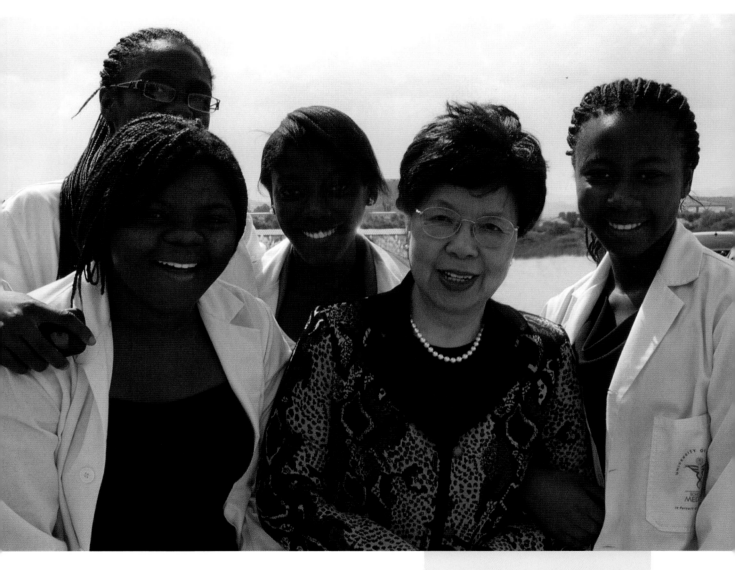

*"We are moving ahead
towards achieving
universal health coverage
with essential health
interventions for neglected
tropical diseases, the
ultimate expression of
fairness."*

Dr Margaret Chan
Director-General
World Health Organization

FOREWORD BY THE DIRECTOR-GENERAL OF THE WORLD HEALTH ORGANIZATION

Much has happened since the World Health Organization (WHO) issued its first report on neglected tropical diseases in 2010. That assessment of the burden caused by these diseases, and of the tools and strategies available for their control, brought cause for general optimism, although specific obstacles to controlling individual diseases were also identified. In January 2012, WHO built on various resolutions and decisions of its governing bodies as well as this previous assessment of opportunities and obstacles – and on the growing sense of optimism – by issuing a roadmap with visionary time-bound goals for controlling, eliminating or eradicating several of these ancient diseases. That ambitious agenda was almost immediately endorsed by the *London declaration on neglected tropical diseases*, which expressed a strong and broad-based will to seize these new opportunities. Commitments on the part of ministries of health in endemic countries, global health initiatives, funding agencies and philanthropists escalated, as did donations of medicines from pharmaceutical companies and the engagement of the scientific community.

With the publication of this report, the control of neglected tropical diseases enters a new phase. Unprecedented recent progress has revealed unprecedented needs for refinements in control strategies, and new technical tools and protocols. The roadmap identified preventive chemotherapy as a key strategy for tackling, often jointly, a number of these diseases. In 2010, 711 million people worldwide received preventive chemotherapy for at least one neglected tropical disease. Since some of these treatments confer protection against three or more diseases, the impact on the total burden of disease is even greater than suggested by this number. The substantial increases in donations of medicines made since the previous report call for innovations that simplify and refine delivery strategies – from forecasting and costing, to the monitoring of drug efficacy and impact, to testing for signs that pathogens are developing resistance under the pressure of mass drug administration. While the prospects for expanding coverage are now vastly improved, endemic countries absorb these donations through large-scale mobilizations of their own, often limited, health resources, further underscoring the need for streamlining and simplification.

The fact that many of these diseases are coendemic emphasizes the need to deliver preventive chemotherapy as an integrated package. Funding for programmes is increasingly provided for the implementation of integrated drug delivery. Campaigns using mass drug administration to target different diseases are now better coordinated, reducing the demands on national capacities and resources. To reduce these demands even further, WHO has developed a package of programmatic tools that facilitate integrated planning and costing, integrate requests for drugs, and simplify and consolidate reporting. In particular, the control of lymphatic filariasis and onchocerciasis are recognized as being intertwined, and calling for closely coordinated programme planning, service delivery and shared indicators for monitoring and evaluation.

FOREWORD

Some needs arise from the sheer magnitude of success. As more programmes approach their milestones and targets, new tools and protocols are needed to assess the intensity of transmission, support decision-making about when mass drug administration can be stopped, and then to verify interruption of transmission. Monitoring vectorial capacity as a proxy for monitoring transmission intensity in humans is an approach that may be far less costly and disruptive to communities. However, it may be necessary to further develop the tools and the capacity for such monitoring.

Some of these diseases, including especially deadly ones like human African trypanosomiasis and visceral Leishmaniasis, remain extremely difficult and costly to manage. Treatments for human African trypanosomiasis have been donated. But the control of Buruli ulcer, Chagas disease and yaws is hampered by imperfect technical tools, although recent developments for yaws look promising. Nonetheless, progress against these especially challenging diseases is being made through the development of innovative and intensive management strategies. Above all, innovations in vector control deserve more attention as playing a key part in reducing transmission and disease burden, especially for dengue, Chagas disease and the Leishmaniases.

Overcoming neglected tropical diseases makes sense both for economies and for development. The prospects for success have never been so strong. Many millions of people are being freed from the misery and disability that have kept populations mired in poverty, generation after generation, for centuries. We are moving ahead towards achieving universal health coverage with essential health interventions for neglected tropical diseases, the ultimate expression of fairness. This will be a powerful equalizer that abolishes distinctions between the rich and the poor, the privileged and the marginalized, the young and the old, ethnic groups, and women and men.

I thank the community of partners for their exceptional commitment and goodwill. We can all be proud of the progress that has been made, step by step over several decades, and that has now swelled into a true pro-poor movement that promises to have a substantial and lasting impact. Through your efforts, the people previously left behind are catching up by a show-case of universal health coverage for control of neglected tropical diseases. By taking these actions, our control efforts will provide convincing evidence of the power of global public health and solidarity.

Dr Margaret Chan
Director-General
World Health Organization

SUMMARY

In January 2012, the World Health Organization (WHO) published a roadmap
(*1*) setting targets for the prevention, control, elimination and eradication of 17
neglected tropical diseases or conditions: Buruli ulcer, Chagas disease, taeniasis/
cysticercosis, dengue, dracunculiasis, echinococcosis, endemic treponematoses,
foodborne trematodiases, human African trypanosomiasis, the Leishmaniases,
leprosy, lymphatic filariasis, onchocerciasis, rabies, schistosomiasis, trachoma and
soil-transmitted helminthiases.

The roadmap marked a major strategic advance since the publication in 2010 of
WHO's first report on neglected tropical diseases (*2*), which set targets for the
eradication of dracunculiasis (2015) and yaws (2020). Furthermore, 6 targets were
set for the elimination of 5 neglected tropical diseases by 2015, and a further 10
elimination targets were set for 2020, either globally or in selected geographical
areas, for 9 neglected tropical diseases (*Annex 3a*). The roadmap also set out targets
for intensified control of dengue, Buruli ulcer, cutaneous Leishmaniasis, selected
zoonoses and helminthiases (*Annex 3b*).

The roadmap inspired the *London declaration on neglected tropical diseases* (*3*), endorsed
by partners and stakeholders in January 2012 who pledged to sustain, expand and
extend control, elimination and eradication programmes to ensure the necessary
supply of medicines and other interventions. The impact and wide dissemination
of the London declaration demonstrate that the global public-health agenda now
embraces neglected tropical diseases.

This second report, *Sustaining the drive to overcome the global impact of neglected tropical
diseases*, further elaborates concepts discussed in the roadmap, describes the need for
sustainable progress, and examines the challenges in implementation encountered by
Member States, WHO and their partners.

The following are highlights of this second report.

- Since 2012, a significant increase in donated medicines has allowed WHO to
  scale up the delivery of preventive chemotherapy.[1] As of 2012, 600 million
  tablets of albendazole or mebendazole became available annually to treat
  school-aged children. Programmes in countries where soil-transmitted
  helminthiases are endemic have already requested an additional 150 million
  tablets – a figure indicative of the significant increase in treatment coverage.
  For schistosomiasis, itis expected that improved access to praziquantel will
  enable an estimated 235 million people to be treated by 2018 (*4*).

---

[1] In this instance, preventive chemotherapy refers to the widespread delivery of quality-
assured, single-dose medicines as preventive treatment against helminthiases and trachoma.

- Impressive progress is being made towards eradicating dracunculiasis; it is estimated that eradication of the disease will yield a 29% increase in economic returns for the agricultural sector of countries where the disease is no longer endemic (5). Heightened community-based surveillance activities, used together with national programmes of integrated disease surveillance and response, are expected to intensify case detection and the subsequent containment of cases, and further reduce transmission in the drive towards eradication. Despite achievements and successes, operational challenges remain in Chad, Ethiopia, Mali and South Sudan.

- WHO's new Morges strategy (6) aims at eradicating yaws by 2020 using a new treatment policy designed to replace those developed in the 1950s, which mainly centred on delivering injections of benzathine benzylpenicillin. Published in January 2012 (7), the findings of a study in Papua New Guinea show that a single dose of oral azithromycin is as effective as intramuscular benzathine benzylpenicillin in treating yaws, thus revitalizing prospects for eradication through the delivery of mass treatment to infected and at-risk populations in the estimated 14 countries where yaws is endemic. This new strategy of treating the entire community overcomes the limitations of penicillin injections, which require trained health-care personnel to deliver case by case treatment.

- This report analyses the opportunities to provide public-health interventions globally after the decisive technical briefing on neglected tropical diseases chaired by the President of the Sixty-fifth World Health Assembly, Her Excellency Professor Thérèse Aya N'dri-Yoman, the Minister of Health of Côte d'Ivoire, in May 2012. Convened at the behest of countries where these diseases are endemic, the meeting noted the "unprecedented force" characterizing the global effort against neglected tropical diseases, and encouraged Member States to increase cooperation with one another and strengthen their political commitment in order to sustain the goals and meet the targets of WHO's roadmap. This report emphasizes the need for national programmes to continue developing a culture of integrated and coordinated planning and programme management to enable programmes to scale up effectively and encourage commitment from governments.

- The work of overcoming neglected tropical diseases builds on five public-health strategies: (i) preventive chemotherapy; (ii) innovative and intensified disease-management; (iii) vector control and pesticide management; (iv) safe drinking-water, basic sanitation and hygiene services, and education; and (v) veterinary public-health services. Although one approach may predominate for the control of a specific disease or group of diseases, evidence suggests that more effective control results when several approaches are combined and delivered locally.

SUMMARY

- In order to measure progress towards the roadmap's targets, this report defines the concepts of elimination and eradication for some neglected tropical diseases and expands that of universal health coverage as it applies to neglected tropical diseases. Universal coverage of prevention and control interventions for neglected tropical diseases depends critically on strong and efficient health systems, access to essential medicines of assured quality at affordable prices, a well-trained and motivated work force, as well as the involvement of sectors other than health, including finance, education, agriculture and veterinary public health, water and sanitation, and environmental management.

- This report discusses the phased implementation of the roadmap, identifies associated challenges, and proposes plans to mitigate some of the challenges. Obstacles and risks to implementation are as diverse as the diseases themselves, and are invariably linked: some include the effects of natural disasters and human conflicts that result in the displacement of millions of people, and disrupt public-health interventions and disease surveillance.

- The transmission and persistence of pathogens responsible for neglected tropical diseases depend on vectors or intermediate hosts. Thus, there is the risk that sufficient access to medicines alone will not enable targets to be achieved if measures to control vectors or their intermediate hosts and species are inadequate. In 2012, dengue ranked as the most important mosquito-borne viral disease with an epidemic potential in the world. There has been a 30-fold increase in the global incidence of dengue during the past 50 years, and its human and economic costs are staggering. The world needs to change its reactive approach and instead implement sustainable preventive measures that are guided by entomological and epidemiological surveillance (*8*).

- Innovative and intensified management for treating diseases that are difficult to diagnose and that cause severe complications requires specific approaches tailored to the features of each disease; to the various forms of infections; to available tools, medicines and technical abilities; and the mobility and readiness of decentralized medical teams to detect patients and manage individual cases. For dengue, Chagas disease, lymphatic filariasis, the Leishmaniases and onchocerciasis – the vector-borne diseases that account for an estimated 16% of the burden of infectious diseases (*9*) – vector control remains key to reducing transmission.

- Sufficient human-resources capacity (both technical and managerial) is required to support the scaling up of interventions at all levels of national health-care systems as well as to mobilize resources. WHO's new Working Group on Capacity Strengthening has been active since December 2012.

SUMMARY

- Notwithstanding global economic constraints, support from Member States and their partners must be expanded to ensure that new products are developed for preventing, diagnosing and controlling these diseases; that services continue to expand; and that much-needed improvements to health systems are made. Expertise in preventing and controlling some neglected tropical diseases, and managing their vectors, will have to be enhanced if the targets set by the World Health Assembly in many resolutions over the years are to be met.

REFERENCES

[1] *Accelerating work to overcome the global impact of neglected tropical diseases: a roadmap for implementation*. Geneva, World Health Organization, 2012 (WHO/HTM/NTD/2012.1).

[2] *Working to overcome the global impact of neglected tropical diseases: first WHO report on neglected tropical diseases*. Geneva, World Health Organization, 2010 (WHO/HTM/NTD/2010.1).

[3] *The London Declaration on Neglected Tropical Diseases* (available at: http://www.unitingtocombatntds. org/endorsements or http://www.unitingtocombatntds.org/downloads/press/london_declaration_on_ntds.pdf; accessed December 2012).

[4] *Schistosomiasis: progress report 2001–2011 and strategic plan 2012–2020*. Geneva, World Health Organization, 2012 (WHO/HTM/NTD/PCT/2012.7).

[5] Jim A, Tandon A, Ruiz-Tiben E. *Cost-benefit analysis of the global dracunculiasis eradication campaign*. Washington DC, World Bank, 1997 (Policy Research Working Paper No. 1835).

Eradication of yaws – the Morges strategy. *Weekly Epidemiological Record*, 2012, 87:189–194.

[7] Mabey D. Oral azithromycin for treatment of yaws. *Lancet*, 2012, 379:295–297.

[8] *Global strategy for dengue prevention and control 2012–2020*. Geneva, World Health Organization, 2012 (WHO/HTM/NTD/VEM/2012.5).

[9] *The global burden of disease: 2004 update*. Geneva, World Health Organization, 2008.

THE GLOBAL PUBLIC-HEALTH AGENDA NOW EMBRACES NEGLECTED TROPICAL DISEASES

Since its founding in 1948, the agenda of the World Health Organization (WHO) has included a commitment to working to reduce the burden of disease that impairs the health and well-being of millions of people living in areas where poverty is prevalent.

1.1 RECENT DEVELOPMENTS IN PREVENTION AND CONTROL

Since its founding in 1948, the agenda of the World Health Organization (WHO) has included a commitment to working to reduce the burden of disease that impairs the health and well-being of millions of people living in areas where poverty is prevalent. The first resolution of the World Health Assembly concerning neglected tropical diseases (NTDs) was adopted in that same year, urging Member States to control the vectors responsible for the transmission of pathogens. Since then, the World Health Assembly has adopted a further 66 resolutions calling on Member States to work to overcome NTDs. Key resolutions aimed at preventing and controlling NTDs are listed in *Annex 1*.

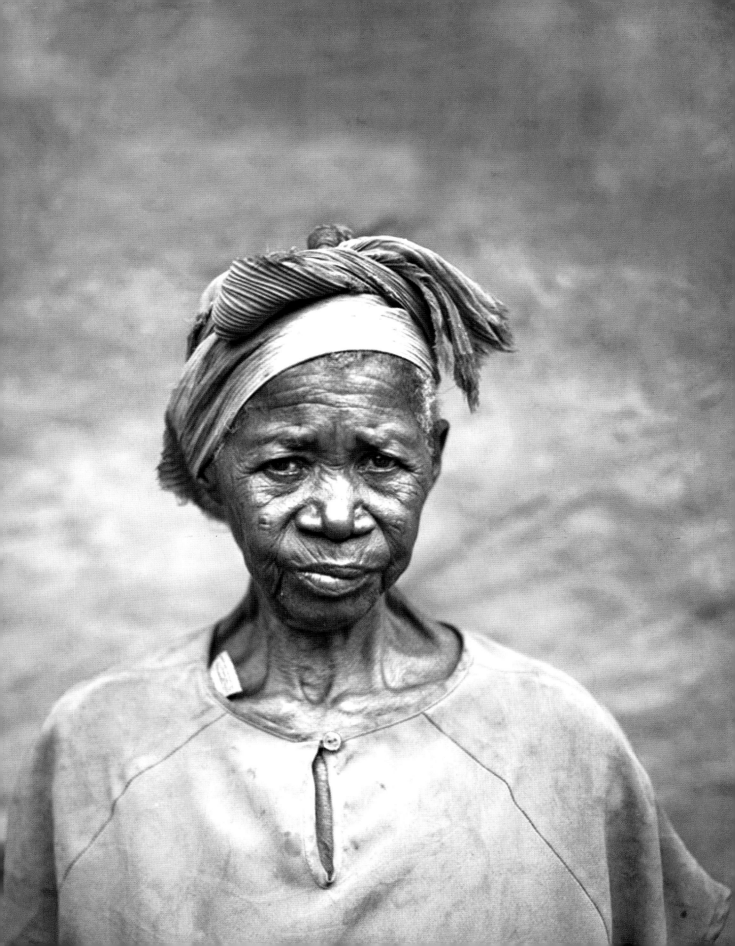

The first WHO report on neglected tropical diseases (the first report) (*1*) described the evolution of the global effort to control 17 NTDs. Nine of these are caused by microparasitic pathogens and eight by macroparasitic pathogens (*2*) that involve vectors, and intermediate and reservoir hosts (*Box 1.1.1*). The pathogens themselves have exceedingly complex life-cycles, population dynamics, infection processes and epidemiologies, causing diverse diseases and pathologies. Their commonality is their persistence and prevalence in people and communities living in poverty and social exclusion.

BOX 1.1.1 Causes of neglected tropical diseases

Microparasitic pathogens	Macroparasitic pathogens
• Buruli ulcer	• Cysticercosis
• Chagas disease	• Dracunculiasis
• Dengue	• Echinococcosis
• Human African trypanosomiasis	• Foodborne trematodiases
• Leishmaniases	• Lymphatic filariasis
• Leprosy	• Onchocerciasis
• Rabies	• Schistosomiasis
• Trachoma	• Soil-transmitted helminthiases
• Treponematoses	

The purpose of this second WHO report on NTDs (the second report) is to sustain the progress that has been made in overcoming their global impact. The report has four objectives:

1. To report on the planning and progress of WHO's recommended public-health strategies for controlling, eliminating and eradicating NTDs;

2. To describe and update the global status of the 17 NTDs discussed in the first report (*1*);

3. To identify action points to ensure the successful implementation of the roadmap as it relates to targets for control, and the need for control activities;

4. To propose how WHO should contribute to expanding control efforts in relation to the roadmap.

The current encouraging position of prevention and control has been reached through the efforts of Member States, WHO and their many partners. The bedrock of much of the effort has been the growing commitments made by the partners that have generously donated medicines (*Annex 2*).

1.2   THE ROADMAP AND THE LONDON DECLARATION

In January 2012, WHO published *Accelerating work to overcome the global impact of neglected tropical diseases: a roadmap for implementation* (the roadmap) (*3*) at a meeting of partners uniting to combat neglected tropical diseases. These partners have been crucial to the successes achieved: they have donated resources, expertise, time and energy to develop, deliver and expand interventions. On 30 January 2012, the partners made a commitment to help overcome NTDs; this commitment is outlined in the *London declaration on neglected tropical diseases* (the London declaration) (*4*) (*Box 1.2.1*). The continuing informal relationships and goodwill that exist among WHO, the community of partners and the governments of endemic countries have been essential to achieving the progress described in this second report.

1.3   OPPORTUNITIES FOR PUBLIC-HEALTH PROGRAMMES

Following dissemination of the London declaration, partners in the NTD community have declared their willingness to fulfil commitments aimed at eradicating NTDs. By honouring their commitments, partners are taking the opportunity to improve the health of millions of people. In addition to the London declaration's optimism, it also includes seven points that highlight actions to be undertaken to reach the roadmap's targets (*Box 1.2.1*). Many of these activities are already under way. For example, efforts are being made to expand access to the increased donations of essential medicines used for preventive chemotherapy. Tools for monitoring and evaluating interventions are being improved.

The call to enhance and ensure efficient collaboration among partners at national and international levels is important if only to avoid duplication of effort. The funding gap should be closed, not only to support research for developing new diagnostics, medicines and vaccines but also to enable countries where these diseases are endemic to expand their capacity and implement national health plans. The funding gap may be the biggest obstacle to reaching the roadmap's targets, given the global economic uncertainty.

On the first day of the Sixty-fifth World Health Assembly in May 2012, at the request of the President of the Assembly, Her Excellency Professor Thérèse Aya N'dri-Yoman, the Minister of Health of Côte d'Ivoire, WHO organized the first ever technical briefing on NTDs. This briefing was an important step towards reaching the goals and targets set in the roadmap. The Sixty-sixth World Health Assembly in May 2013 will consider how Member States can best overcome the global impact of NTDs.

BOX 1.2.1 The London Declaration on Neglected Tropical Diseases

UNITING TO COMBAT NEGLECTED TROPICAL DISEASES

Ending the Neglect & Reaching 2020 Goals

▶ **Endorsers:**

Abbott

AstraZeneca

Bayer

Becton Dickinson

Bill & Melinda Gates Foundation

Bristol-Myers Squibb

CIFF

DFID

DNDi

Eisai

Gilead

GlaxoSmithKline

Johnson & Johnson

Lions Clubs International

Merck KGaA

MSD

Mundo Sano

Novartis

Pfizer

Sanofi

USAID

World Bank

LONDON DECLARATION ON NEGLECTED TROPICAL DISEASES

▶ *For decades, partners including pharmaceutical companies, donors, endemic countries and non-government organisations have contributed technical knowledge, drugs, research, funding and other resources to treat and prevent Neglected Tropical Diseases (NTDs) among the world's poorest populations. Great progress has been made, and we are committed to build on these efforts.*

Inspired by the World Health Organization's 2020 Roadmap on NTDs, we believe there is a tremendous opportunity to control or eliminate at least 10 of these devastating diseases by the end of the decade. But no one company, organization or government can do it alone. With the right commitment, coordination and collaboration, the public and private sectors will work together to enable the more than a billion people suffering from NTDs to lead healthier and more productive lives – helping the world's poorest build self-sufficiency. As partners, with our varied skills and contributions, **we commit to doing our part to:**

- Sustain, expand and extend programmes that ensure the necessary supply of drugs and other interventions to help **eradicate** Guinea worm disease, and help **eliminate** by 2020 lymphatic filariasis, leprosy, sleeping sickness (human African trypanosomiasis) and blinding trachoma.

- Sustain, expand and extend drug access programmes to ensure the necessary supply of drugs and other interventions to help **control** by 2020 schistosomiasis, soil-transmitted helminthes, Chagas disease, visceral leishmaniasis and river blindness (onchocerciasis).

- Advance R&D through partnerships and provision of funding to find next-generation treatments and interventions for neglected diseases.

- Enhance collaboration and coordination on NTDs at national and international levels through public and private multilateral organisations to work more efficiently and effectively together.

- Enable adequate funding with endemic countries to implement NTD programmes necessary to achieve these goals, supported by strong and committed health systems at the national level.

- Provide technical support, tools and resources to support NTD-endemic countries to evaluate and monitor NTD programmes.

- Provide regular updates on the progress in reaching the 2020 goals and identify remaining gaps.

To achieve this ambitious 2020 vision, we call on all endemic countries and the international community to join us in the above commitments to provide the resources necessary across sectors to remove the primary risk factors for NTDs—poverty and exposure—by ensuring access to clean water and basic sanitation, improved living conditions, vector control, health education, and stronger health systems in endemic areas.

We believe that, working together, we can meet our goals by 2020 and chart a new course toward health and sustainability among the world's poorest communities to a stronger, healthier future.

1.4   COSTS OF EXPANDING ACTIVITIES

This second report demonstrates that interventions have expanded rapidly; and detailed plans for further expansion are being prepared based on the progress made to date.

A priority for planning is to address the cost of expanding implementation activities. It is important to consider the size of the funding gap that will have to be closed if the roadmap's targets are to be achieved. Accurate evidence-based costings must be obtained for the interventions that will be necessary to meet the targets in the roadmap. Robust costing will help governments, donors and partners to see how their contributions are helping to close the funding gap.

WHO is undertaking the necessary analysis and making appropriate forecasts. This process will be monitored by the Strategic and Technical Advisory Group for Neglected Tropical Diseases, and the results should be published by 2014.

1.5   WHO AND THE ROADMAP'S TARGETS

WHO has a pivotal role in leading the work that must be undertaken if the challenges in the roadmap are to be met, and the targets and milestones reached. Since 2008, the Strategic and Technical Advisory Group for Neglected Tropical Diseases and its specialist working groups have provided advice to WHO. At each meeting, the advisory group agrees a series of action points for WHO to address in addition to its ongoing work; these action points are communicated by the Chair of the advisory group to the Director-General.

The following action points take into consideration some of the advisory group's recommendations (more are available from the report of the meeting held in April 2012) (5) as well as input from WHO regions and countries; these responses illustrate how WHO addresses the action points with the aim of ensuring that the roadmap's targets are met.

- Scale up preventive chemotherapy: (i) seek to embed the culture of integrated and coordinated planning and management of preventive chemotherapy among disease-specific programmes; (ii) assist national programmes in scaling up; and (iii) encourage governments' commitments.

- Organize planning for the integrated and coordinated scaling down of programmes once targets are reached and sustained.

- Promote practical definitions for eradication and elimination in the context of NTD targets. Assist countries in setting quantifiable definitions for control of a specific disease and ensure that definitions relate to the prevailing epidemiology in endemic countries.

- Identify and disseminate a single measurable indicator for each NTD targeted for eradication, elimination or control in the roadmap.

- Improve the planning for, forecasting for and regularity of the supply of medicines by using appropriate coordination mechanisms among donation programmes.

- Take the lead in establishing active reporting on the efficacy and safety of medicines against human African trypanosomiasis, the Leishmaniases and Chagas disease.

- Circulate the draft manual for schoolteachers who are involved in distributing anthelminthic medicines to a larger number of partners to seek input from a wide range of stakeholders, and take into account the need to produce local versions in national or local languages.

- Establish a global rabies-control strategy for dogs and humans.

- Form a coordination group to engage in advance planning for the global prevention and control of dengue.

REFERENCES

[1] *Working to overcome the global impact of neglected tropical diseases: first WHO report on neglected tropical diseases*. Geneva, World Health Organization, 2010 (WHO/HTM/NTD/2010.1).

[2] Anderson RM, May RM. *Infectious diseases of humans: dynamics and control*. Oxford, Oxford University Press, 1991.

[3] *Accelerating work to overcome the global impact of neglected tropical diseases: a roadmap for implementation*. Geneva, World Health Organization, 2012 (WHO/HTM/NTD/2012.1).

[4] *Table of commitments*. London, Uniting to Combat NTDs, 2012 (http://www.unitingtocombatntds. org/downloads/press/ntd_event_table_of_commitments.pdf ; accessed December 2012).

[5] *Report of the WHO Strategic and Technical Advisory Group for Neglected Tropical Diseases 24–25 April 2012*. Geneva, World Health Organization, 2012 (http://www.who.int/entity/neglected_ diseases/NTD_STAG_Report_2012.pdf; accessed November 2012).

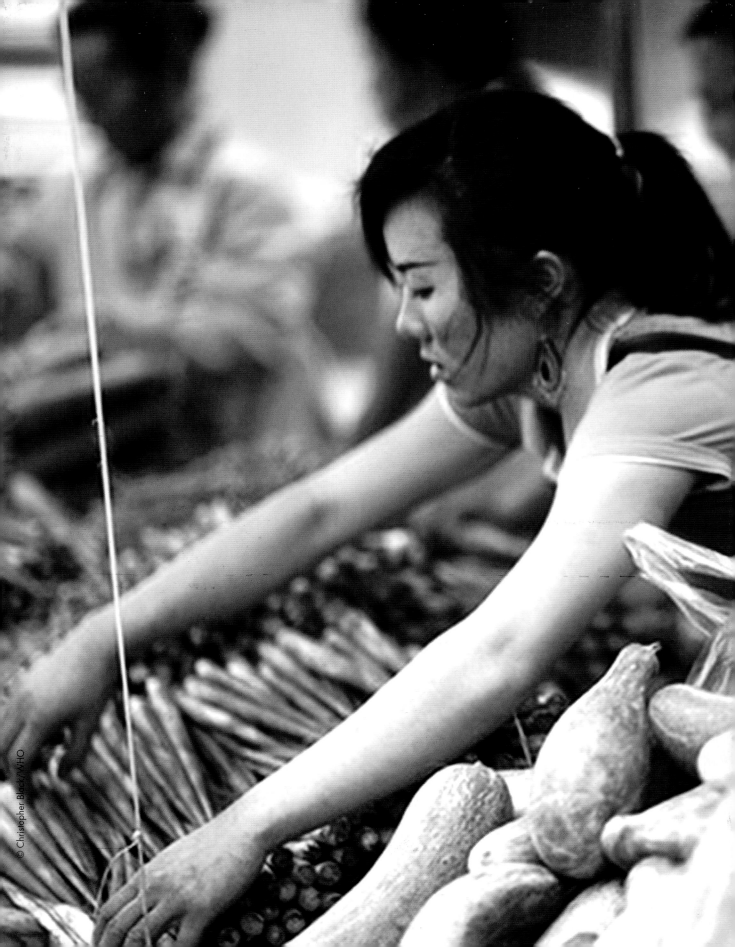

REACHING THE ROADMAP'S TARGETS

The roadmap set targets for eradicating dracunculiasis by 2015 and eradicating endemic treponematoses (yaws) by 2020. Furthermore, 6 elimination targets for 5 NTDs have been set for 2015, and a further 10 targets for the elimination of 9 NTDs by 2020.

The roadmap (*1*) set targets for eradicating dracunculiasis by 2015 and eradicating endemic treponematoses (yaws) by 2020. Furthermore, 6 elimination targets for 5 NTDs have been set for 2015, and a further 10 targets for the elimination of 9 NTDs by 2020 (*Annex 3a*). Some of the elimination targets are global, some are regional and some are country-specific. Some NTDs are targeted in more than one location. For example, onchocerciasis is targeted for elimination in Latin America and Yemen by 2015, and in selected African countries by 2020. The roadmap also sets out a matrix of targets for intensifying control efforts against dengue, Buruli ulcer, cutaneous Leishmaniasis and various helminthiases (*Annex 3b*); these control targets are variable and include validation of strategies, pilot projects, vector control and expansion of preventive chemotherapy, again in a variety of locations.

Of major importance is the need for consensus on the use of the terms eradication, elimination and control in the context of the roadmap. Consensus is essential for ensuring that communication about targets is clear and for ensuring agreement that a target has been reached.

2.1   PRACTICAL DEFINITIONS OF ERADICATION, ELIMINATION AND CONTROL

After consulting with the Strategic and Technical Advisory Group for Neglected Tropical Diseases in 2012 (*2*), WHO recommended that the following definitions should be used for the roadmap's targets.

Eradication is the permanent reduction to zero of the worldwide incidence of infection caused by a specific pathogen as a result of deliberate efforts, with no risk of reintroduction. In some cases a pathogen may become extinct, but others may be present in confined settings, such as laboratories.

Elimination (interruption of transmission) is the reduction to zero of the incidence of infection caused by a specific pathogen in a defined geographical area as a result of deliberate efforts; continued actions to prevent re-establishment of transmission may be required.

Control is the reduction of disease incidence, prevalence, intensity, morbidity, or mortality, or a combination of these, as a result of deliberate efforts. The term "elimination as a public-health problem" should be used only upon achievement of measurable targets for control set by Member States in relation to a specific disease. Continued intervention measures may be required to maintain this reduction.

By December 2012, a single measurable indicator was recommended to be used for each disease targeted in the roadmap for eradication, elimination or control (*Annex 4*). Ideally, confirmation of eradication and elimination requires independent assessment; Member States have requested that WHO establish certification processes for smallpox, poliomyelitis and dracunculiasis (*3,4*).

2.2   OBSTACLES AND RISKS TO ACHIEVING TARGETS

Prospects for achieving the roadmap's targets will be improved if obstacles and risks are identified and assessed so that mitigating plans can be implemented. Some problems may be intractable, but others might be avoided; accepting their existence now may be helpful later if WHO and its partners in the NTD community need to review circumstances that may have delayed the achievement of targets. Obstacles and risks to implementation do not stand in isolation but will invariably be linked – for example, vector control and pesticide resistance – and will vary among countries and diseases.

2.2.1   Conflicts and population displacement

Natural disasters and violent human conflicts lead to the death and displacement of millions of people who, as a result, suffer from disease, as well as starvation and sexual and physical abuse (5). Since 1945, some 23 conflicts have been waged or continue to be waged in countries in sub-Saharan Africa, where NTDs are prevalent (6). Since 1998, 5.4 million people have died in the Democratic Republic of the Congo, and 1.5 million have become refugees or been displaced. In 2011, the total global number of refugees was estimated to be about 10.5 million; in 2010, the total number of internally displaced persons was about 27.5 million, with 11.5 million of these being in Africa (7).

Armed conflict is likely to disrupt the delivery of preventive chemotherapy, and adequate case management and disease surveillance, put the lives of health workers at risk, and impede access to treatment. Plans can be made to reach refugees and internally displaced persons, especially if they are living in camps. The numbers may seem relatively small compared with those requiring preventive chemotherapy but, in addition to their health needs, displaced persons may serve as reservoirs of infection or agents of dispersal when national borders are porous.

2.2.2   Population growth

By 31 October 2012, the world's population had reached 7 billion, with most of the growth occurring once again in the countries where NTDs are prevalent (8). Population growth is predicted to continue to be greatest in sub-Saharan Africa, which includes 33 of the 49 countries considered to be least developed according to social and economic indicators (9). The population in sub-Saharan Africa is currently 840 million; with a likely annual increase of 20 million, the population will be 1.02 billion by 2020. This is the year set to meet 1 eradication target, 4 global elimination targets and 10 regional or country-based elimination targets (*Annex 3a*). This projected population growth should be considered to ensure that resources will be available to deliver sufficient treatments.

2.2.3   Vector control

The transmission and persistence of many pathogens – such as those responsible for dengue, Chagas disease, foodborne trematodiases, human African trypanosomiasis, Leishmaniases, dracunculiasis, lymphatic filariasis, onchocerciasis and schistosomiasis – depend on vectors or intermediate hosts. There is a risk that sufficient access to medicines alone will not achieve a specific target if measures to control vectors or intermediate hosts are inadequate. More efforts need to be made to deal with vectors and the chemicals involved in their control.

Vector control relies mainly on the use of pesticides. Sound management of pesticides requires collaboration among sectors for agriculture, health and the environment. WHOPES (the WHO Pesticide Evaluation Scheme) works in collaboration with the FAO (the Food and Agriculture Organization of the United Nations) and UNEP (the United Nations Environment Programme); it continues to serve as the main resource for information on pesticide management, and provides guidance on the safety, quality control, application and efficacy of pesticides.

2.2.4   Resistance to medicines and pesticides

Resistance to a medicine or pesticide is defined as a loss of susceptibility to that medicine or pesticide in a population that was previously sensitive to the appropriate therapeutic dose or controlling application. Veterinary use of anthelminthics to control nematode infections in sheep has led to the selection of populations resistant to albendazole, mebendazole, levamisole, pyrantel and ivermectin (*10*). In mice experimentally infected with a human isolate of *Schistosoma mansoni* and exposed to repeated doses of praziquantel, evidence has shown that praziquantel-resistant genes are present in the isolate (*11*).

There is no solid evidence of resistance in pathogens responsible for human helminthiases, despite the enormous number of treatments for NTDs that have been delivered over many years using a small number of medicines. This artificial selection pressure, however, enhances the risk of inducing strains of medicine-resistant pathogens. The shorter a pathogen's generation time, the more likely it is that resistance will emerge. In anticipation of the development of such resistance, especially with the scaling up of preventive chemotherapy, WHO's Strategic and Technical Advisory Group for Neglected Tropical Diseases has established a working group to monitor the efficacy of medicines, and prepare standard operating procedures to detect resistance early (*12*).

It is equally important to prepare procedures and alternative strategies that can be used if resistance is detected.

2.2.5   Insufficient capacity for scaling up

Projections for the progressive scaling up of interventions en route towards 2020 and the related milestones, assume that necessary resources will become available as required. In terms of human resources, this implies that technical and managerial capacity will be built at all levels of national health-care systems so that simultaneous nationwide implementation can be carried out and maintained for as long as necessary as part of the delivery of routine health-care interventions, similar to the ways that nationwide vaccination programmes were introduced. If adequate sustainable capacity is not built into national health plans and strategy, it is unlikely that such a large number of endemic countries will simultaneously be able to scale up their programmes. Significant resources are required to ensure that programmes are fully implemented, milestones are reached, and then programmes are scaled down. It is unlikely that these resources will be generated entirely from external sources, thus consistent efforts to mobilize national resources from various sectors will need to be made in endemic countries. The worldwide private sector has made unprecedented pledges to supply the medicines required for large-scale distribution, but such external support needs adequate domestic infrastructure. The impact of programmes will need to be monitored, and adjustments may need to be made to implementation strategies to reach the roadmap's targets in the most cost-effective manner.

2.2.6   Expectations overtaking science

Evidence from clinical trials and community studies demonstrates that individual treatment and the large-scale delivery of effective chemotherapy reduces and controls morbidity caused by NTDs. However, current scientific information may not be sufficient to underpin all aspects of NTD control. For example, a key assumption guiding most programmes is that a given number of treatments or rounds of mass drug administration will interrupt transmission in all settings, whether transmission occurs from person to person or through vectors or their intermediate hosts. Information collected by monitoring coverage and evaluating the impact of strategies will help validate this assumption and refine control strategies.

2.2.7   Inadequate support for research

Fundamental research and operational research will continue to be essential components in the work to overcome NTDs. In 2012, WHO's Special Programme for Research and Training in Tropical Diseases published its *Global report for research on infectious diseases of poverty* (*13*). This comprehensive report recognized that research into NTDs lags behind research into the diseases that affect more affluent people. The report called for more equitable support for research into NTDs to increase knowledge about these diseases and to improve control interventions. The strategies used to combat NTDs are based on science. Research must continue if these diseases are to be overcome.

2.2.8   Climate change

Climate change is now accepted as resulting mainly from an increase in the emissions of greenhouse gases (water vapour, carbon dioxide, methane, nitrous oxide) released as a result of human activity. By the end of the 21st century, the earth's temperature may rise above mid-1990 levels by 1.1 °C to 6.4 °C, a change that is predicted to lead to additional heat waves, floods and droughts. The World Meteorological Organization and WHO have jointly published the *Atlas of health and climate* (*14*), which explores the numerous and variable effects of climate change on infectious diseases, including NTDs. The effects of climate change on populations of vectors and on the persistence and transmission of NTDs are of particular concern.

REFERENCES

[1]   *Accelerating work to overcome the global impact of neglected tropical diseases: a roadmap for implementation.* Geneva, World Health Organization, 2012 (WHO/HTM/NTD/2012.1).

[2]   *Report of the WHO Strategic and Technical Advisory Group for Neglected Tropical Diseases, Geneva, 24–25 April 2012.* Geneva, World Health Organization, 2012 (http://www.who.int/entity/neglected_diseases/NTD_STAG_Report_2012.pdf; accessed November 2012).

[3]   *Resolution WHA42.29: elimination of dracunculiasis.* Geneva, World Health Organization, 1989.

[4]   *Resolution WHA44.5: eradication of dracunculiasis.* Geneva, World Health Organization, 1991.

[5]   *Violence and health in the WHO African Region.* Brazzaville, WHO Regional Office for Africa, 2010.

[6]   Hawkins V. *Stealth conflicts: how the world's worst violence is ignored.* Burlington, VT, Ashgate Publishing Company, 2008

[7]   *UNHCR global trends 2011: a year of crises.* Geneva, Office of the United Nations High Commissioner for Refugees, 2011.

[8]   *State of world population 2012. By choice, not by chance: family planning, human right and development.* New York, NY, United Nations Population Fund, 2012.

[9]   *World development report 2011: conflict, security and development.* Washington, DC, World Bank, 2011.

[10]   Mansour TE. *Chemotherapeutic targets in parasites: contemporary strategies.* Cambridge, Cambridge University Press, 2002.

[11]   Cioli D. Praziquantel: is there real resistance and are there alternatives? *Current Opinion in Infectious Diseases*, 2000, 13:659–663.

REACHING THE ROADMAP'S TARGETS

[12] *Report of the third meeting of the Global Working Group on monitoring the efficacy of drugs for neglected tropical diseases, 13–14 February 2012*. Geneva, World Health Organization, 2012.

[13] *Global report for research on infectious diseases of poverty*. Geneva, World Health Organization on behalf of the Special Programme for Research and Training in Tropical Diseases, 2012.

[14] *Atlas of health and climate*. Geneva, World Health Organization and World Meteorological Organization, 2012.

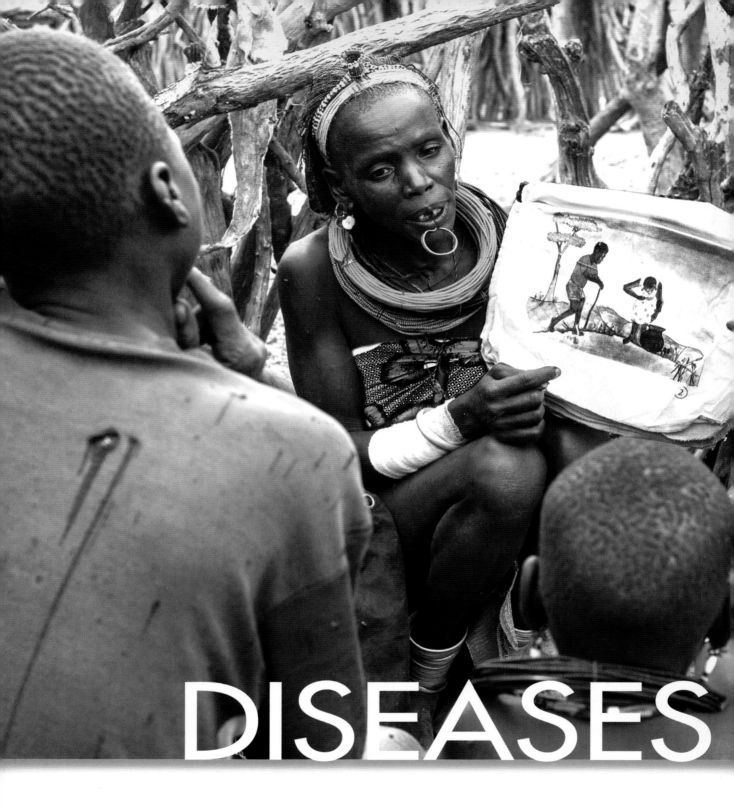

DISEASES

This second report is mainly concerned with assessing the progress made in preventing and controlling NTDs in relation to the targets and milestones in the roadmap. This report also includes updated information on the distribution and impact of NTDs and their effects on women and children.

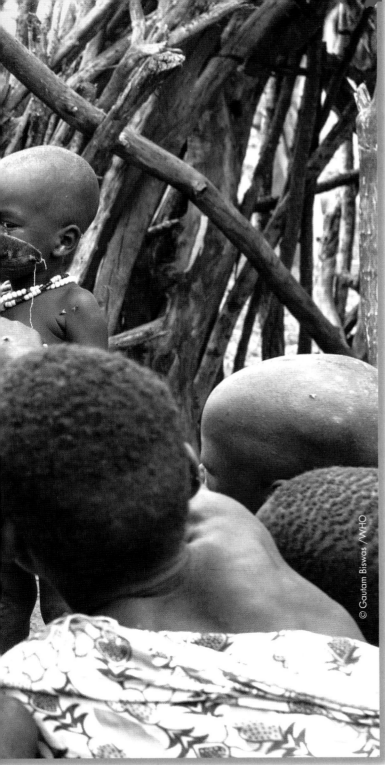

A volunteer in South Sudan teaches children how to avoid guinea-worm infection.

The number of dracunculiasis cases reported to WHO worldwide has decreased steadily, with 542 cases in 2012.

WHO published a detailed account of the distribution and impact on public health of 17 NTDs in its first report in 2010 (*1*) and updated the report in 2011 (*2*). This second report is mainly concerned with assessing the progress made in preventing and controlling NTDs in relation to the targets and milestones in the roadmap (*3*). This report also includes updated information on the distribution and impact of NTDs and their effects on women and children.

The latest WHO estimates of several NTDs remain those published in its 2004 update of *The global burden of disease*

(*4*). However, the results of a 2010 study by the Institute for Health Metrics and Evaluation includes updated estimates for many NTDs. These estimates have not yet been endorsed by WHO, but WHO will hold an expert consultation in February 2013 on the significance of the results. In addition, WHO is preparing a regional update of deaths by cause, which will be released in early 2013.

REFERENCES

[1] *Accelerating work to overcome the global impact of neglected tropical diseases: a roadmap for implementation.* Geneva, World Health Organization, 2012 (WHO/HTM/NTD/2012.1).

[2] *Working to overcome the global impact of neglected tropical diseases: first WHO report on neglected tropical diseases. Update 2011.* Geneva, World Health Organization, 2011 (WHO/HTM/NTD/2011.3).

[3] *Accelerating work to overcome the global impact of neglected tropical diseases: a roadmap for implementation.* Geneva, World Health Organization, 2012 (WHO/HTM/NTD2012.1).

[4] *The global burden of disease: 2004 update.* Geneva, World Health Organization, 2008.

WOMEN, CHILDREN AND NEGLECTED TROPICAL DISEASES

Many NTDs disproportionately affect women and children. Those living in remote areas are most vulnerable to infections, and their biological and sociocultural consequences. Deliberate global health responses are needed to promote interventions in the biological and social contexts in which these diseases persist. Additional efforts are required to collect epidemiological data that show the differential impact of these diseases according to a patient's sex and age in order to better inform policies, and guide targeted interventions for sustainable control.

Biological consequences

The contribution of biological sex and age to the outcomes of infections can be significant. For example, the combined effects of puberty and first pregnancy in young mothers can reactivate leprosy. Nerve damage from leprosy is accelerated in pregnant and lactating women, 45% of whom develop silent neuritis, including those on chemotherapy and those considered cured (*1*).

An estimated 44 million pregnant women are infected with hookworm at any one time, including up to one third of all pregnant women in sub-Saharan Africa (*2*). Hookworm infection contributes to approximately 7% of the 20% of maternal deaths in Africa caused by anaemia. Schistosomiasis affects an estimated 10 million pregnant women in Africa alone, half of whom consequently develop anaemia and its complications during pregnancy (complications include increased maternal morbidity, low birth weight and other adverse outcomes) (*3*). Hookworm infection and schistosomiasis contribute to infertility and a range of problems that adversely affect female reproductive health. Women who have urogenital schistosomiasis are three times to four times more likely to become infected with HIV (*4*).

Children are vulnerable to infections because of their immature immune systems and exposure through daily activities, such as playing, assisting with farming activities and living in substandard, overcrowded conditions. About one third of the world's population are infected with soil-transmitted helminths: this includes more than 270 million preschool-aged children and more than 600 million school-aged children living in areas where these parasites are intensively transmitted (*5*). Sequelae include stunted growth, impaired cognitive function, limited educational advancement and compromised future economic prospects (*6*).

Yaws affects children (mostly boys) aged 2–14 years; they account for 75% of all reported cases and in turn serve as the main reservoirs of infection (*7*). Trachoma occurs mostly in young children; they are the reservoirs of infection and are predisposed to developing blindness later in life (*8*). Congenital (mother-to-child) transmission of Chagas disease occurs in about 1–10% of cases, which can lead to clinical manifestations from birth and even the possibility of transmission to second generations (*9*). Visceral Leishmaniasis can also be transmitted to fetuses by their mothers (*10*). The development of dengue haemorrhagic fever and dengue shock syndrome, and secondary-type antibody response, are affected by age and sex; the incidences are higher in young children and females than in males, particularly in Asia (*11*).

Sociocultural consequences

Women living in endemic areas are often exposed to these diseases during domestic activities that place them in regular contact with vector habitats, such as while collecting water. Dracunculiasis transmission in Nigeria is influenced by daily life and coping mechanisms at household and community levels (*12*). Of the 1058 cases reported in 2011, 349 of those infected were women and 411 were children; these women and children represented 72% of all cases reported in 2010 (*13*).

Child-rearing places women in close contact with small children – the main reservoir of *Chlamydia trachomatis* infection – and makes them three to four times more likely to develop blinding trachoma than men (*14*). Studies from Egypt and Sudan show a complex relationship between schistosomiasis and sex in relation to domestic activities and farming (*15*). There is accumulating evidence of a sex-specific negative impact of emerging zoonotic pathogens on women's health. For all zoonotic illnesses – particularly disabling and wasting conditions, and mental conditions, such as those associated with neurocysticercosis – women are called upon to devote a disproportionately large share of their time to caring for sick members of their family, both at home and when seeking or receiving treatment outside the home (*16*).

Stigma

During the past half century, social stigma has become increasingly recognized as an important social determinant of the effectiveness of disease control, mainly through its effect on health-seeking behaviour and adherence to treatment, especially for women. Women consistently experience longer delays before beginning treatment for visceral Leishmaniasis than men (5 months for women versus 3 months for men in Bangladesh) (*17*). Cutaneous Leishmaniasis causes painful, unsightly long-lasting skin lesions and leaves permanent, disfiguring scars on the face or arms. Women are particularly stigmatized by scarring: they are considered unacceptable for marriage, sometimes by their own families; they are often forcefully separated from their children during the illness, not allowed to breastfeed, and may suffer mental illness as a result (*18*).

Lymphatic filariasis disfigures and onchocerciasis blinds, stigmatizing entire communities; consequently, women may find it difficult to marry and the morbidity caused by their impairment interferes with their earning capacity (*19*). Although disfigurement and social stigmatization are not lethal, they may cause or precipitate psychological disorders and restrict social participation. NTDs affect not only women's physical well-being but also their psychological, social and economic health. The potential burden of mental illness, particularly depressive illness, has recently been highlighted (*20*). The number of individuals who suffer from disabling and stigmatizing conditions suggests that mental illness may be an additional, previously unrecognized burden of NTDs (*21*).

REFERENCES

[1] Duncan ME, Pearson JM. Neuritis in pregnancy and lactation. *International Journal of Leprosy and Other Mycobacterial Diseases*, 1982, 50:31–38.

[2] Empowering women and improving female reproductive health through control of neglected tropical diseases. *PLoS Neglected Tropical Diseases*, 2009, 3(11)e559 (doi:10.1371/journal.pntd.0000559).

[3] Friedman JF et al. Schistosomiasis and pregnancy. *Trends in Parasitology*, 2007, 23:159–164; King C et al. Transmission control for schistosomiasis – why it matters now. *Trends in Parasitology*, 2006, 22:575–582; Nour NM. Schistosomiasis: health effects on women. *Reviews in Obstetrics and Gynecology*. 2010, 3:28–32.

[4] Kjetland EF et al. Female genital schistosomiasis due to *Schistosoma haematobium*: clinical and parasitological findings in women in rural Malawi. *Acta Tropica*, 1996, 62:239–255; Downs JA et al. Urogenital schistosomiasis in women of reproductive age in Tanzania's Lake Victoria region. *American Journal of Tropical Medicine and Hygiene*, 2011, 83:364–369.

[5] *Neglected tropical diseases: PCT databank*. Geneva, World Health Organization, 2010 (http://www.who.int/neglected_diseases/preventive_chemotherapy/databank/en/; accessed November 2012).

[6] Solomons NW. Pathways to the impairment of human nutritional status by gastrointestinal pathogens. *Parasitology*, 1993, 107(Suppl.):S19–S35; Crompton DWT, Nesheim MC. Nutritional impact of intestinal helminthiasis during the human life cycle. *Annual Review of Nutrition*, 2002, 22:35–59; Curtale F et al. Intestinal helminths and xerophthalmia in Nepal: a case-control study. *Journal of Tropical Pediatrics*, 1995, 41:334–337; Stephenson LS et al. Physical fitness, growth and appetite of Kenyan school boys with hookworm, *Trichuris trichiura* and *Ascaris lumbricoides* infections are improved four months after a single dose of albendazole. Journal of Nutrition, 1993, 123:1036–1046; Callender JE et al. Growth and development four years after treatment for the Trichuris dysentery syndrome. *Acta Paediatrica*, 1998, 87:1247–1249; Stephenson LS, Latham MC, Ottesen EA. Malnutrition and parasitic helminth infections. *Parasitology*, 2000, 121(Suppl.):S23–S38; Nokes C et al. Parasitic helminth infection and cognitive function in school children. *Proceedings of Biological Sciences*, 1992, 247:77–81; Kvalsvig JD, Cooppan RM, Connolly KJ. The effects of parasite infections on cognitive processes in children. *Annals of Tropical Medicine and Parasitology*, 1991, 85:551–568; Miguel E, Kremer M. *Identifying impacts on education and health in the presence of treatment externalities*. Cambridge, MA, National Bureau of Economic Research, 2001 (Working paper 8481).

[7] Asiedu K, Sherpbier R, Raviglione M, eds. *Buruli ulcer*: Mycobacterium ulcerans *infection*. Geneva, World Health Organization Global Buruli Ulcer Initiative, 2000 (WHO/CDS/CPE/GBUI/200.1).

[8] Barenfanger J. Studies on the role of the family unit in the transmission of trachoma. American *Journal of Tropical Medicine and Hygiene*, 1975, 24:509–515.

[9] Schenone H et al. Congenital Chagas disease of second generation in Santiago, Chile. Report of two cases. *Revista do Instituto de Medicina Tropical de São Paulo*, 2001, 43:231–232.

[10] Isam A et al. Congenital kala-azar and leishmaniasis in the placenta. *American Journal of Tropical Medicine and Hygiene*, 1992, 46:57–62.

[11] Cobra C et al. Symptoms of dengue fever in relation to host immunologic response and virus serotype, Puerto Rico, 1990–1991. *American Journal of Epidemiology*, 1995,142:1204–1211; Pinheiro FP, Corber SJ. Global situation of dengue and dengue haemorrhagic fever, and its emergence in the Americas. *World Health Statistics Quarterly*, 1997, 50:161–169; *Dengue haemorrhagic fever: diagnosis, treatment and control*. Geneva, World Health Organization, 1986:7–15.

[12] Watts SJ, Brieger WR, Yacoob M. Guinea worm: an in-depth study of what happens to mothers, families and communities. *Social Science and Medicine*, 1989, 29:1043–1049.

[13] Dracunculiasis eradication: global surveillance summary, 2011. *Weekly Epidemiological Record*, 2012, 87:177–188.

[14] Frick KD, Mecaskey JW. Resource allocation to prevent trachomatous low vision among older individuals in rural areas of less developed countries. *Documenta Ophthalmologica*, 2002, 105:1–21.

[15] Michelson, EH. Adam's rib awry? Women and schistosomiasis. *Social Science and Medicine*. 1993, 37:493–501; Feldmeier H et al. Female genital schistosomiasis: new challenges from a gender perspective. *Tropical and Geographical Medicine*. 1995, 47(Suppl. 2):S2–S15.

[16] Theiler RN et al. Emerging and zoonotic infections in women. *Infectious Disease Clinics of North America*, 1998, 22:755–772; R. Theiler, 2008, Hotez PJ 2008, Wiess MG 2008, WHO 2006.

[17] Indu B et al. Visceral leishmaniasis: consequences to women in a Bangladeshi community. *Journal of Women's Health*, 2004, 13:360–364.

[18] Kassi M et al. Marring leishmaniasis: the stigmatization and the impact of cutaneous leishmaniasis in Pakistan and Afghanistan. *PLoS Neglected Tropical Diseases*, 2008, 2(10):e259 (doi:10.1371/journal.pntd.0000259);Reithinger R et al. Social impact of leishmaniasis, Afghanistan. *Emerging Infectious Diseases*. 2005, 11:634–636.

[19] Coreil J, Mayard G, Addis D. *Support groups for women with lymphatic filariasis in Haiti*. Geneva, World Health Organization, 2003; Bandyopadhyay L. Lymphatic filariasis and the women of India. *Social Science and Medicine*, 1996, 42:1401–1410; Person B et al. Health-related stigma among women with lymphatic filariasis from the Dominican Republic and Ghana. *Social Science and Medicine*, 2009, 68:30–38; Vlassoff C et al. Gender and the stigma of onchocercal skin disease in Africa. *Social Science and Medicine*, 2000, 50:1353–1368.

[20] Molyneux DH. The 'Neglected Tropical Diseases': now a brand identity; responsibilities, context and promise. *Parasites and Vectors*, 2012, 5:23.

[21] Litt et al. Neglected tropical diseases and mental health: a perspective on comorbidity. *Trends in Parasitology*, 2012, 28:195–201.

3.1   DENGUE

Introduction

Dengue is a mosquito-borne viral disease of public-health significance affecting all regions of WHO. The flavivirus is transmitted mainly by female *Aedes aegypti* mosquitoes and, to a lesser extent, by female *A. albopictus* mosquitoes. Between 1955 and 1959, the number of countries reporting cases of dengue increased from three to eight; in 2012, the geographical distribution of dengue included more than 125 countries. This increase underscores the need to implement sustainable prevention and control interventions rather than rely on responses to outbreaks. The emergence and spread of the four dengue viral serotypes across WHO's African, the Americas, South-East Asia and the Eastern Mediterranean regions represents a pandemic threat. Although the full global burden of the disease is uncertain, the patterns are alarming both for human health and the global economy (*1*) (*Fig.3.1.1*).

Fig. 3.1.1 Global distribution of countries or areas at risk of dengue transmission, 2011

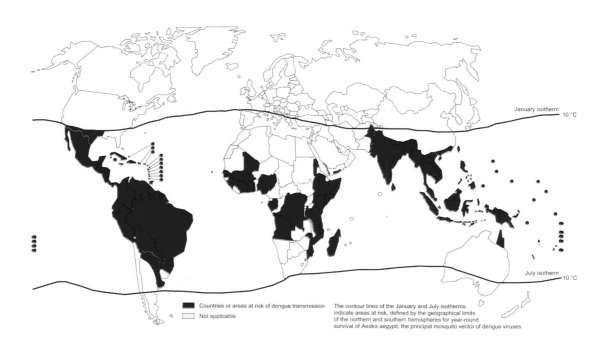

Countries or areas at risk of dengue transmission

Not applicable

The contour lines of the January and July isotherms indicate areas at risk, defined by the geographical limits of the northern and southern hemispheres for year-round survival of *Aedes aegypti*, the principal mosquito vector of dengue viruses

Distribution

During 1960–2010 in the African Region, 22 countries reported sporadic cases or outbreaks of dengue; 12 additional countries reported that dengue was restricted to travellers. The presence of disease and the high prevalence of antibodies to dengue virus in serological surveys suggest that endemic dengue virus infection exists in all or many parts of Africa. Dengue may be underreported in Africa owing to a lack of awareness among health-care providers, the presence of other febrile illnesses (especially malaria), and insufficient testing and reporting that hinders systematic surveillance.

Dengue is regarded as an emerging disease in WHO's Eastern Mediterranean Region since reporting to WHO of laboratory-confirmed cases in this region has been occurring for only two decades. Generally, cases have been detected along the coasts of countries bordering the Red Sea and the Arabian Sea, and in Pakistan. The current situation of dengue in countries of the region can be stratified as follows.

- **Group A: Pakistan, Saudi Arabia and Yemen** – Dengue is emerging as a major public-health problem in this group. During the past two decades (1990–2010), repeated outbreaks have occurred in urban centres and the disease has spread to rural areas in Pakistan and Yemen. An outbreak in Lahore in 2011 caused more than 300 deaths.

- **Group B: Djibouti, Somalia, and Sudan**– Outbreaks are becoming more frequent; multiple virus serotypes are cocirculating; and the disease is probably expanding its geographical reach in these countries.

- **Group C: Oman** – Imported cases of dengue have been reported, but there is no evidence of endemicity or local transmission.

- **Group D** – This includes countries where dengue has not yet been reported, although the inability of a surveillance system to detect the disease cannot be ruled out.

In much of the Region of the Americas interruption in transmission resulted from the campaign to eradicate *A. aegypti* during the 1960s and early 1970s. However, vector surveillance was not sustained so mosquitoes thrived and dengue outbreaks recurred in the Caribbean, and in Central America and South America (2). The region is now in a hyperendemic state, with indigenous transmission occurring in almost all countries. A regional initiative uses an integrated management strategy for prevention, and this offers the most promising approach to disease control (3).

Dengue is endemic in WHO's South-East Asia Region, although there is significant variation in incidence among countries and within each country. The seasonal pattern of dengue differs among countries: in India, the number of cases peaks between August and November; in Indonesia it peaks in January and February; and in Myanmar and Sri Lanka, the peak occurs between May and August. Severe dengue is endemic in most of the countries in the South-East Asia Region (*4*).

During the 1990s in WHO's European Region, *A. albopictus* rapidly became established, mainly through the global trade in used tyres. The threat of dengue outbreaks exists in Europe. In 2010, local transmission of the virus was reported for the first time in Croatia and France; imported cases were detected in several other European countries. An outbreak of dengue was also reported from Madeira island of Portugal recently (2012).

Although the number of reported dengue cases in the Western Pacific Region fell to around 50 000 annually in 1999 and 2000 after an epidemic in 1998, the incidence of dengue has increased during the past decade. In 2010, the region reported 353 907 cases, including 1073 deaths (case-fatality rate, 0.30%). The incidence of dengue was highest in the Lao People's Democratic Republic, but most cases and deaths were reported from the Philippines. Island nations have been susceptible to epidemics: in 2011 both Micronesia and the Marshall Islands had epidemics. Increases in the number of cases reported from Malaysia and Singapore indicate sustained epidemic activity.

Impact

Fig. 3.1.2 shows the number of deaths from dengue reported to WHO by Member States from 2006 to 2010. There has been a steady rise in the number of cases of dengue and severe dengue reported during 1955–2010 (*Fig. 3.1.3*).

Fig. 3.1.2 Number of deaths from dengue reported to WHO by Member States, 2006–2010

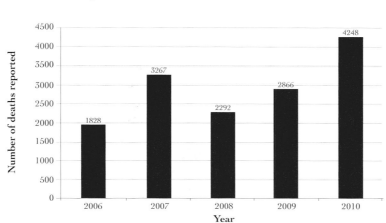

Fig. 3.1.3 Average number of cases of dengue and severe dengue reported
to WHO annually during 1955–2007 compared with the number
of cases reported during 2008–2010 (2011 data are incomplete)

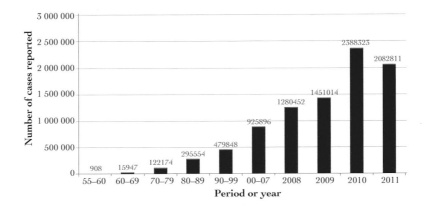

Strategy (roadmap targets and milestones)

The objectives of the Global strategy for dengue prevention and control, 2012–2020 (5) are by
2020 to reduce mortality from dengue by at least 50% and reduce morbidity by
at least 25% using 2010 as the baseline (*Annex 3b*). The strategy has five technical
elements: (i) diagnosis and case management; (ii) integrated surveillance and outbreak
response; (iii) sustainable vector control; (iv) future vaccine implementation; and (v)
basic operational and implementation research.

Table 3.1.1 shows proposed indicators for monitoring and evaluating the performance
and impact of dengue prevention and control efforts; assessing these efforts should
contribute to achieving the targets and milestones in the roadmap.

REFERENCES

[1] *Atlas of health and climate*. Geneva, World Health Organization and World Meteorological
Organization, 2012 (http://www.who.int/globalchange/publications/atlas/report/en/index.
html; accessed November 2012).

[2] *Plan continental de ampliación e intensificación del combate al Aedes aegypti. Informe de un grupo de trabajo,
Caracas, Venezuela. Abril 1997 [Continental plan of expansion and intensification of the fight against
Aedes aegypti. Report of a working group, Caracas, Venezuela. April 1997]*. Washington, DC, Pan
American Health Organization, 1997.

[3] San Martin JL et al. The epidemiology of dengue in the Americas over the last three decades:
a worrisome reality. *American Journal of Tropical Medicine and Hygiene*, 2010, 82:128–135.

[4] *Comprehensive guidelines for prevention and control of dengue and dengue haemorrhagic fever: revised and
expanded edition*. New Delhi, WHO Regional Office for South-East Asia, 2011.

[5] *Global strategy for dengue prevention and control, 2012–2020*. Geneva, World Health Organization,
2012 (WHO/HTM/NTD/VEM/2012.5).

DISEASES

Table 3.1.1 Proposed indicators for monitoring progress in implementing dengue prevention and control efforts

Intended outcome	Indicator	Type			Limitations of the indicator for monitoring and evaluation	Source of data needed to assess the indicator
		Process	Outcome	Impact		
Sustainable control interventions established in 10 endemic countries considered to be priorities	No of countries with dengue programme		√		Quality of services cannot be fully assessed	National report
	No. of countries with strategy for managing insecticide resistance	√			Quality of implementation cannot be assessed	National report
	No. of countries with national strategic and implementation plans for integarted vector management	√			Quality and level of implementation cannot be assessed	National report
Control and surveillance established in all regions	No. of countries and regions reporting dengue data to WHO		√		Quality to ensure true estimates of burden cannot be assessed	National report
	No. of regional initiatives for cross-border sharing of information		√		Full collaboration due to political sensitivities cannot be ascertained	National and regional reports
Morbidity reduction	No. of clinical cases (probable)			√	True burden cannot be ascertained	National and regional reports
	No. of confirmed cases			√	Not all cases may be confirmed	National and regional reports
	No. of severe cases			√	–	National and regional reports
	No. of countries that have reduced dengue morbidity by 25% and mortality by 50%		√		Accuracy of reports	National and regional reports
	Incidence rate			√	Accuracy of estimate of population at risk	National and regional reports
Mortality reduction	No. of confirmed deaths from dengue			√	Lack of proper audit	National and regional reports
	Case-fatality rate			√	–	National and regional reports

3.2   RABIES

Introduction

Rabies is a vaccine-preventable viral disease. However, once symptoms develop, rabies is almost always fatal to humans unless they promptly receive post-exposure prophylaxis. Success in preventing and controlling rabies in humans has been mostly achieved in North America, western Europe, and in a number of Asian and Latin American countries through the implementation of sustained campaigns to immunize and humanely manage dog populations, and to provide post-exposure prophylaxis to people who have been exposed to suspect rabid dogs and other susceptible animals. WHO promotes a wider use of the intradermal route for pre- and post-exposure prophylaxis, which reduces volume and the cost of cell-cultured vaccine by 60–80% (*1*). Raising awareness of the disease among populations at risk, particularly children, is crucial for its elimination. Several countries in Asia and Latin America have developed plans and defined target dates for eliminating human rabies of canine origin (*2–6*).

Fig. 3.2.1 Global distribution of risk to humans of contracting rabies, 2011

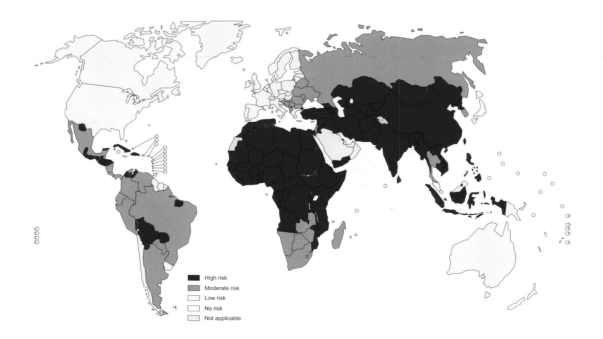

High risk
Moderate risk
Low risk
No risk
Not applicable

Distribution

Rabies causes tens of thousands of human deaths annually worldwide (*7–10*). Its global distribution has changed little since 2010, and most deaths still occur in WHO's African, South-East Asia and Western Pacific regions (*Fig. 3.2.1*). Only a few countries (mainly islands and peninsulas) are rabies-free. Wild mammalian species, including bats, maintain and transmit the virus, but the number of human rabies deaths associated with wildlife is small compared with that following contacts with rabid dogs.

Dog rabies and human rabies transmitted by dogs have been eliminated in many Latin American countries, including Chile, Costa Rica, Panama, Uruguay, and most of Argentina, the states of Sao Paulo and Rio de Janeiro in Brazil, and large parts of Mexico and Peru (*11*). Human rabies transmitted by dogs remains widespread in Cuba, the Dominican Republic, El Salvador, Guatemala, Haiti and the Plurinational State of Bolivia (*12*). Rabies in dogs is actively controlled at the Bolivian–Peruvian border, and in Haiti.

China, Thailand and Sri Lanka continue to report progress in their control activities (*Fig. 3.2.2*). Improvements in control have also been reported from parts of the Philippines, where pilot projects are under way. Sri Lanka aims to eliminate human rabies by 2016 and rabies in dogs by 2020. Indonesia has reported a worsening epidemiological situation: since the end of the 1990s, the disease has emerged in an increasing number of formerly rabies-free islands including Bali (*13,14*).

Fig. 3.2.2 Impact of mass dog vaccination on incidence of human rabies, Sri Lanka, 1970–2010

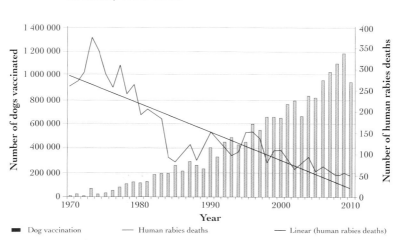

During the past decade, few large-scale dog vaccination campaigns against rabies have been implemented in Africa, where the disease continues to be largely uncontrolled. Notable exceptions are the national dog rabies control programmes under way in Morocco and Tunisia, and large-scale projects carried out in parts of the United Republic of Tanzania and South Africa, particularly in the province of KwaZulu-Natal (*15*). Recent surveys have indicated the extremely limited availability of post-exposure prophylaxis, one of the most important causes of rabies deaths, in most of sub-Saharan Africa. In-depth country-specific studies show that official reports may underestimate rabies incidence by more than 100-fold, because most deaths occur in communities rather than in hospitals (*16,17*), and those that occur in hospitals are frequently misdiagnosed for other encephalitis (*18*). Neural tissue-based vaccines are still used for post-exposure prophylaxis in Algeria and Ethiopia. Although rabies is endemic in both the Middle East and central Asia, there is very little information available on its true impact on human and animal health (*19,20*).

Human rabies transmitted by vampire bats is a public-health issue of increasing importance in Latin America, particularly in remote areas of the Amazon region of Brazil, Colombia, Ecuador and Peru (*21*), where exposed populations do not have access to appropriate care. In addition, climate change may lead to an expansion of the geographical distribution of these bats and associated zoonoses (*22*).

Impact

Several unpublished studies have reported high levels of uncertainty about estimates of mortality owing to a lack of accurate primary data. Methods have been developed to improve the accuracy of determining mortality attributable to rabies. A predictive approach that uses a probability decision-tree method has been introduced to establish the likelihood of developing rabies following a bite from a dog suspected to be rabid. This approach has been used to estimate mortality from rabies in Africa and Asia (*16*) and, more recently, applied to determine country-specific mortality estimates in Bhutan (*23*) and Cambodia (*24*).

During the past decade, China and India have remained major contributors to the rabies burden, accounting for 25–40% of global mortality from the disease depending on the source and time of the estimate (*16,25*). The number of clinically diagnosed deaths from rabies reported to the Chinese centre for disease control (*26*) rose from 150 in 1996 to 3300 in 2007, and then fell to 1917 rabies deaths in 2011. The number of infected counties has, however, remained almost stable since 2008 (*Fig. 3.2.3*).

In India, the rabies situation has improved over the past 10 years since the use of outdated vaccines has ended, and they have been replaced with modern vaccines; these changes have been coupled with improvements in the accessibility of post-exposure

DISEASES

prophylaxis (*27*). Measures to curb dog reproduction (using animal birth control) and rabies-control activities together have contributed to reducing the circulation of the virus in the dog population (*28, 29*) (*Fig. 3.2.4*). A large-scale verbal autopsy survey estimated there were 12 700 human deaths from rabies in India in 2005.

Fig. 3.2.3 Number of human deaths from rabies and number of counties reporting rabies, China, 2000–2011[a]

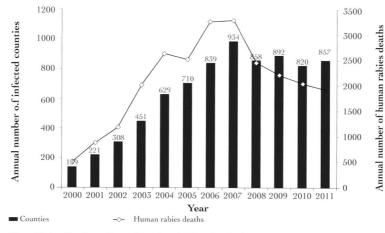

* Source: Weizhong Yang, Deputy Director, Chinese Center for Disease Control and Prevention

Fig. 3.2.4 Number of human deaths from rabies, Chennai, India since beginning the animal birth control programme, 1996–2010

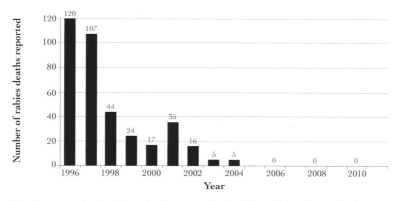

* Source: Except where otherwise noted, the numbers of cases were provided by the Ministry of Health and Family Welfare, Government of Tamil Nadu; the number for 2003 was provided by the Corporation of Chennai; the number for 2004 was provided by Dr K. Manivasan, Deputy Commissioner (Health), Chennai Corporation; the number for 2008 was provided by Dr B. Kuganatham, Health Officer, Chennai Corporation.

Strategy (roadmap targets and milestones)

Although progress has been made at the international and national levels in breaking the cycle of rabies neglect through assertive advocacy, much remains to be done in promoting the use of existing tools and strategies to eliminate this disease from entire WHO regions.

WHO, the FAO, the World Organisation for Animal Health (OIE) and the Global Alliance for Rabies Control are collaborating to eliminate human rabies of canine origin (*30*). By 2015, human rabies transmitted by dogs should have been eliminated, and dog to dog transmission should have been stopped in all Latin American countries (*2,3*). An expert consultation organized by the WHO's Regional Office for South-East Asia in 2011 provided a regional strategic framework for eliminating human rabies transmitted by dogs (*31*). The target is to eliminate the disease in endemic South-East Asian countries in the region by 2020, and to certify and then maintain this status. The first part of the strategic plan covers the 5-year period 2012–2016, and should reduce by half the current number of human deaths estimated to have been caused by rabies.

The ASEAN Plus Three countries (the Association of Southeast Asian Nations plus China, Japan and the Republic of Korea) have agreed to take steps towards eliminating rabies by 2020 (*5*). A regional ASEAN framework on preventing and controlling the disease was developed in 2009 and endorsed by the working group on livestock in 2010; it is being updated.

REFERENCES

[1]   Rabies vaccines: WHO position paper. W*eekly Epidemiological Record*, 2010, 85:309–320.

[2]   *15th Inter-American meeting, at the ministerial level, on health and agriculture. Rio de Janeiro, Brazil, 11–12 June 2008*. Washington, DC, Pan American Health Organization, 2007 (RIMSA15/1, Rev. 2 (Sp.).

[3]   *Resolution CD49.R9: elimination of neglected diseases and other poverty-related infections*. Washington, DC, Pan American Health Organization, 2009 (Forty-ninth Directing Council). http://new. paho.org/hq/index.php?option=com_content&task=view&id=2372&Itemid=1967.

[4]   *Strategic framework for elimination of human rabies transmitted by dogs in the South-East Asia Region*. New Delhi, WHO Regional Office for South-East Asia, 2012.

[5]   *Call for action: towards the elimination of rabies in the ASEAN Member States and the Plus Three Countries*. Jakarta, Association of Southeast Asian Nations, 2008.

[6]   *Report of the ASEAN/FAO/OIE/WHO rabies workshop. Chiang Mai, Thailand, 19–20 January 2012*. Jakarta, ASEAN Secretariat, 2012.

[7]   Knobel DL et al. Re-evaluating the burden of rabies in Africa and Asia. *Bulletin of the World Health Organization*, 2005, 83:360–368.

[8]   *WHO Expert Consultation on Rabies: first report*. Geneva, World Health Organization, 2005.(WHO Technical Report Series, No. 931).

[9]   Suraweera W et al. Deaths from symptomatically identifiable furious rabies in India: a nationally representative mortality survey. *PLoS Neglected Tropical Diseases*, 2012, 6(10):e1847 (doi:10.1371/journal.pntd.0001847).

[10] Foreman KJ et al. Modeling causes of death: an integrated approach using CODEm. *Population Health Metrics*, 2012;10:1 (doi:10.1186/1478-7954-10-1).

[11] Schneider MC et al. Current status of human rabies transmitted by dogs in Latin America. *Cadernos de Saúde*, 2007, 23:2049–2063.

[12] *Eliminación de la rabia humana transmitida por perros en América Latina: análisis de la situación* [Elimination of human rabies transmitted by dogs in Latin America: situation analysis]. Washington, DC, Pan American Health Organization, 2005.

[13] Windiyaningsih C et al. The rabies epidemic on Flores Island, Indonesia (1998–2003). *Journal of the Medical Association of Thailand*, 2004, 87:1389–1393.

[14] Agung Gde Putra A. Progress of rabies elimination programme in Bali, Indonesia. In: Sudarshan SN, Ravish HS, eds. *3rd international conference on Rabies in Asia (RIA) Foundation: conference proceedings*. Karnataka, India, Rabies in Asia Foundation, 2011:39–45 (http://www.rabiesinasia.org/riacon2011.html; accessed December 2012).

[15] *Report of the fourth meeting of the International Coordinating Group of the Bill & Melinda Gates Foundation–World Health Organization project on eliminating human and dog rabies. Cebu City, Philippines, 2–4 October 2012*. Geneva, World Health Organization, 2013 (WHO/NTD/NZD/2013.1).

[16] Cleaveland S et al. Estimating human rabies mortality in the United Republic of Tanzania from dog bite injuries. *Bulletin of the World Health Organization*, 2002, 80:304–310.

[17] Hampson CK et al. Rabies exposures, post-exposure prophylaxis and deaths in a region of endemic canine rabies. *PLoS Neglected Tropical Diseases*, 2008, 2:e339 (doi:10.1371/journal.pntd.0000339).

[18] Mallewa DM et al. Rabies encephalitis in malaria-endemic area, Malawi, Africa. *Emerging Infectious Diseases*, 2007, 13:136–139.

[19] *Report of the WHO (HQ-MZCP)/OIE Inter-country expert workshop on protecting humans from domestic wildlife rabies in the Middle East. Amman, Jordan, 23–25 June 2008* (available at www.oie.int/doc/ged/D6490.PDF; accessed January 2013).

[20] *Report of the second meeting of the Middle East and Eastern Europe Rabies Expert Bureau (MEEREB). Paris, France, 5–8 June 2012* (http://www.meereb.info/meetings-concrete-actions; accessed January 2013).

[21] Schneider MC et al. Rabies transmitted by vampire bats to humans: an emerging zoonotic disease in Latin America? *Revista Panamericana Salud Publica*, 2009, 25:260–269.

[22] Mistry S, Moreno A. Modeling changes in vampire bat distributions in response to climate change: implications for rabies in North America. In: *International Conference on Rabies in the Americas*. Atlanta, GA, Centers for Disease Control and Prevention (http://www.rita2009.org/pdf/RITA_XIX_ProgramBook.pdf; accessed 23 October 2012).

23   Tenzin et al. Dog bites in humans and estimating human rabies mortality in rabies endemic areas of Bhutan. *PLoS Neglected Tropical Diseases*, 2011, 5(11):e1391 (doi:10.1371/journal.pntd.0001391).

24   Ly S et al. Rabies situation in Cambodia. *PLoS Neglected Tropical Diseases*, 2009, 3(9):e511 (doi:10.1371/journal.pntd.0000511).

25   Sudarshan M et al. Assessing the burden of human rabies in India: results of a national multi-center epidemiological survey. *International Journal of Infectious Diseases*, 2007, 11:29–35.

26   Yang W. *Epidemiology and prevention of human rabies in China* [Presentation]. CPMA national conference on rabies, Beijing, China, 17–18 May 2012.

27   Goswani A. A clinician overview of the changes in the rabies scenario of India in the last 25 years [Presentation]. *14th National Conference of the Association for Prevention and Control of Rabies in India (APRICON), Kolkata, India, 7–8 July 2012.*

28   Reece JF, Chawla SK. Control of rabies in Jaipur, India, by the sterilisation and vaccination of neighbourhood dogs. *Veterinary Record*, 2006, 159:379–383.

29   Chinny Krishna S. Role of various stakeholders in rabies control [Presentation]. *14th National Conference of the Association for Prevention and Control of Rabies in India* (APRICON), Kolkata, India, 7–8 July 2012.

30   Lembo T et al. Renewed global partnerships and redesigned roadmaps for rabies prevention and control. *Veterinary Medicine International*, 2011, 2011: 923149 (doi:10.4061/2011/923149).

31   *Report on informal consultation to finalize regional strategic framework for elimination of human rabies transmitted by dogs in the South-East Asia Region: Bangkok, Thailand 13–14 June 2011.* New Delhi, WHO Regional Office for South-East Asia, 2012 (SEA-CD-251).

3.3   TRACHOMA

Introduction

Trachoma, caused by infection with *Chlamydia trachomatis*, accounts for about 3% of all cases of blindness worldwide. An estimated 325 million people live in endemic areas: more than 21 million have active trachoma, 7.2 million need surgery for trichiasis, and 1.2 million have become irreversibly blind (*1,2*). In hyperendemic areas, as much as 90% of preschool-aged children may be infected (*3*).

Distribution

Blinding trachoma is hyperendemic in many of the poorest and most remote rural areas in 53 countries in Africa, Asia, Central America and South America, Australia and the Middle-East (*Fig. 3.3.1*) (*1*).

Overall, Africa is the most badly affected continent: 18.2 million cases of active trachoma (85.3% of all cases globally) and 3.2 million cases of trichiasis (44.1% of all cases globally) occur in 29/46 countries in WHO's African Region. The highest

Fig. 3.3.1 Global distribution of trachoma, 2010

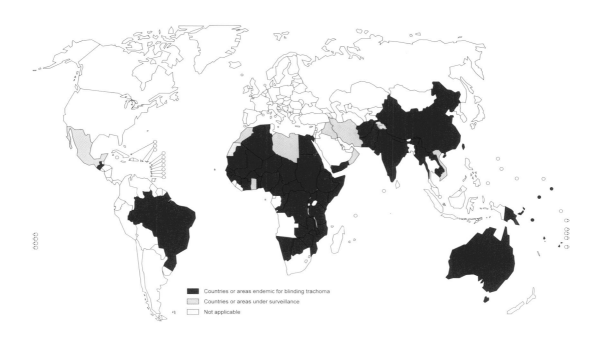

Countries or areas endemic for blinding trachoma
Countries or areas under surveillance
Not applicable

prevalences of active trachoma have been reported from Ethiopia and South Sudan, where the infection often occurs in more than 50% of children who are younger than 10 years; trichiasis is found in up to 19% of adults.

Impact

In addition to blindness, trichiasis and conjunctival scarring, trachoma causes severe ocular pain every time a person blinks (*3,4*). In rural communities in sub-Saharan Africa, an increased mortality rate was found among blind people compared with sighted controls (*5,6*). The annual economic cost of trachoma in terms of lost productivity is estimated to be between US$ 2.9 billion and US$ 5.3 billion, increasing to US$ 8 billion when trichiasis is included (*7*).

Strategy (roadmap targets and milestones)

In 1998, the World Health Assembly resolved to eliminate blinding trachoma as a public-health problem by 2020 (*8*), mainly by implementing the SAFE strategy. This strategy comprises Surgery for individuals with trachomatous trichiasis; Antibiotics to reduce the reservoir of chlamydial infection; Facial cleanliness to reduce the risk of disease transmission; and Environmental improvements that include the safe management of animal and human excreta, promotion of living conditions that reduce ocular promiscuity (that is, unhygienic behaviours such as sharing washcloths used to clean eyes) and crowding, and access to safe water and sanitation facilities (*8,9*). The overall cost effectiveness of implementing the SAFE strategy has been estimated at US$ 54 per case of visual impairment prevented (*10,11*).

Most countries have set target dates for eliminating blinding trachoma, and have agreed with partners to accelerate implementation of the SAFE strategy (*Fig. 3.3.2*).

National data indicate that about 45 million people were treated for trachoma in 2010, and 52 million in 2011, mainly using azithromycin plus tetracycline eye ointment.

The Islamic Republic of Iran, Morocco and Oman have reached elimination targets (known as the ultimate intervention goal, or UIG). In 2011, Ghana, the Gambia and Myanmar achieved their UIGs, and started implementing or planning post-treatment surveillance. Mexico started work in 2011 to verify results of post-treatment surveillance and to identify whether there is a need for further interventions. China confirmed its intention to reach the elimination target by 2016. Brazil has started interventions aimed at eliminating the disease, treating 50 000 people in 2011 and carrying out epidemiological assessments in the Amazonas state. Guatemala organized a national workshop in March 2012 to review the epidemiology of the disease and develop a plan for elimination. Cameroon, the Central African Republic,

Fig. 3.3.2 Target dates set by Member States for eliminating blinding trachoma[a]

2005–2008	2010	2011	2012	2013	2014	2015	2016	2018	2020
Iran(Islamic Republic of)	Ghana	Gambia		Viet Nam	Mauritania	Brazil	Burundi	Central African Republic	Australia
Morocco	Myanmar	Oman			Nepal	Burkina Faso	China		Cameroon
					Pakistan	Cambodia	Côte d'Ivoire		Egypt
						Democratic Republic of the Congo			Ethiopia
									Guinea
						Eritrea			Guinea-Bissau
						Guinea			Kenya
						Lao People's Democratic Republic			Malawi
									Mozambique
									Nigeria
						Mali			Solomon Islands
						Niger			South Sudan
						Senegal			United Republic of Tanzania
									Uganda
									Yemen
									Zambia

No date set for Afghanistan, Chad, Djibouti, Guatemala, India, and Sudan.

■ Achieved   ■ Not confirmed in 2012 Trachoma   ■ New date set
                       Elimination Monitoring Form

[a] Source: Adapted from Trachoma Elimination Monitoring Form

Chad, Ethiopia, Kenya, South Sudan and Zambia organized national workshops in 2011 and 2012 to enable them to respond to the roadmap's targets before or by 2020. In 2011, the Ministry of Health in the Solomon Islands established the post of national trachoma coordinator; mass administration of azithromycin will begin in 2013. The Australian Government[1] is to review guidelines for the public-health management of trachoma, thereby supporting trachoma-control programmes in the country.

REFERENCES

[1] Global WHO Alliance for the Elimination of Blinding Trachoma by 2020: progress report on elimination of trachoma, 2010. *Weekly Epidemiological Record*, 2012, 87:161–168.

[2] Pascolini D, Mariotti SP. Global estimates of visual impairment: 2010. *British Journal of Ophthalmology*, 2011:300539 (doi:10.1136/bjophthalmol-2011-300539).

[3] West SK et al. The epidemiology of trachoma in central Tanzania. *International Journal of Epidemiology*, 1991, 20:1088–1092.

[4] Mariotti SP, Pascolini D, Rose-Nussbaumer J. Trachoma: global magnitude of a preventable cause of blindness. *British Journal of Ophthalmology*, 2009, 93:563–568 (doi:10.1136/bjo.2008.148494).

[1] Refers to the National Trachoma Surveillance and Reporting Unit, Office of Aboriginal and Torres Strait Islander Health, Communicable Diseases Network Australia.

5 Frick KD et al. Trichiasis and disability in a trachoma-endemic area of Tanzania. *Archives of Ophthalmology*, 2001, 119:1839–1844.

6 Kirkwood B et al. Relationships between mortality, visual acuity and microfilarial load in the area of the Onchocerciasis Control Programme. *Transactions of the Royal Society of Tropical Medicine and Hygiene*, 1983, 77:862–868.

7 Courtright P et al. Trachoma and blindness in the Nile Delta: current patterns and projections for the future in the rural Egyptian population. *British Journal of Ophthalmology*, 1989, 73:536–540.

8 *Global elimination of blinding trachoma*. Geneva, World Health Organization, 1998 (Resolution WHA51.11).

9 Frick KD, Hanson CL, Jacobson GA. Global burden of trachoma and economics of the disease. *American Journal of Tropical Medicine and Hygiene*, 2003, 69:1–10.

10 West ES et al. Risk factors for postsurgical trichiasis recurrence in a trachoma-endemic area. *Investigative Ophthalmology and Visual Science*, 2005, 46:447–453.

11 Evans TG et al. Cost-effectiveness and cost utility of preventing tachomatous visual impairment: lessons from 30 years of trachoma control in Burma. *British Journal of Ophthalmology*, 1996, 80:880–889.

3.4   BURULI ULCER

Introduction

Buruli ulcer is a chronic necrotizing skin disease caused by infection with *Mycobacterium ulcerans*; historically, the disease has been reported from 33 countries, of which 15 countries report cases annually (*1*). Globally, there is no clear pattern in the distribution of cases, but a trend towards an increase has been found in Australia, Gabon and Ghana (*2,3,4,5*).

Distribution

The 33 countries where Buruli ulcer has been detected mainly have tropical and subtropical climates (*6*) (*Fig. 3.4.1*). In 2011, cases were reported from about half of these countries, and most of the countries reporting cases are in Africa, where efforts to control the disease have been focused during the past decade. About 5000 cases annually are reported from 15/33 countries, but this number is thought to be low (*Fig. 3.4.2*). The incidence in endemic regions of Ghana has been estimated at 150 cases/100 000 population (*7*). Japan has reported 32 cases since 1980 (*8*), and

Fig. 3.4.1 Global distribution of Buruli ulcer, 2011

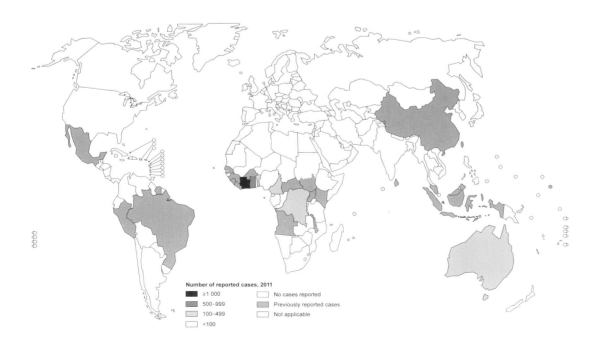

Number of reported cases, 2011
- ≥1 000
- 500–999
- 100–499
- <100
- No cases reported
- Previously reported cases
- Not applicable

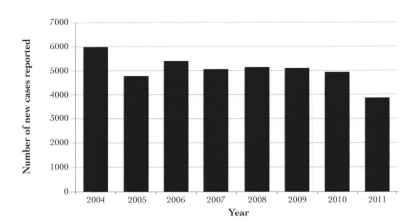

Fig. 3.4.2   Global number of new cases of Buruli ulcer reported to WHO,
2004–2011

Australia reported 520 cases between 2002 and 2011, where a trend towards an increase is evident (*4,9*). An increase in the number of cases has also been seen in Gabon (*2*); but in Benin since 2007 the number of cases has been decreasing (*9*).

The data available to WHO are limited for three reasons: (i) within endemic countries, control activities have a restricted geographical scope, and data may not reflect the national burden; (ii) there are areas where only a few activities or no activities are occurring, and so the extent of the disease is not known; (iii) underreporting may be caused by insufficient knowledge of the disease and the fact that it affects mainly poor, rural communities.

Impact

The main problems associated with Buruli ulcer are the long periods needed for healing, a process that includes hospitalization, and the contractures resulting from late healing, especially when lesions cross joints and treatment is inadequate. At least 25% of healed cases have some degree of disability (*3,10*). Death in patients is related to sepsis and tetanus (*11*). Coinfection with HIV is an emerging issue for which optimal clinical management has still to be defined (*12,13*).

In Ghana during 2001–2003, the median annual total cost of the disease to a household ranged from US$ 76 (16% of a work year) per patient with a lesion to US$ 428 (89% of a work year) per patient who had undergone amputation (*14*). The average cost of treating a case was estimated to be US$ 780 per patient during 1994–1996, an amount exceeding per capita government spending on health (*10*). This economic pattern has also been reported from Australia, Cameroon and Gabon (*2,15,16*).

Strategy (roadmap targets and milestones)

Members of the Global Buruli Ulcer Initiative include academic and research institutions, donor agencies, nongovernmental organizations, Member States and WHO. The aims of the initiative are to raise awareness, improve access to early diagnosis and treatment, and promote the development of better tools for treatment and prevention. The strategy, based on the declaration on Buruli ulcer adopted in Cotonou, Benin, in 2009 (*17*), is designed to minimize morbidity and disability through early detection and treatment (*Table 3.4.1*). Opportunities to implement control measures for Buruli ulcer together with other public-health programmes should not be missed.

Table 3.4.1 Components of the Buruli ulcer control strategy

• **Community-level activities**	• **Strengthening of the health system**
– Ensure early case-detection at the community level using trained village volunteers	– Improve infrastructure, equipment and logistics (use decentralized health centres)
– Provide information, education and communication campaigns in communities and schools	– Train health workers
– Train village-based health workers and strengthen community-based surveillance systems	– Use standardized recording and reporting forms BU 01 and BU 02, and map affected communities
• **Standardized case management**	• **Supportive activities**
– Ensure laboratory confirmation of cases	– Supervise, monitor and evaluate control activities
– Treat with antibiotics	– Advocate, engage in social mobilization and develop partnerships
– Provide wound care	– Conduct operational research
– Provide surgery	
– Prevent disability and provide rehabilitation	

In 2004, WHO published guidelines recommending treatment with a combination of antibiotics (rifampicin and streptomycin) (*1,9,18*); since then, nearly 40 000 people have benefited from combination antibiotic therapy, which has almost halved the need for surgery, the mainstay of treatment in the past (*19*). The roadmap's first target for achieving intensified control of Buruli ulcer requires completion by 2015 of a clinical trial of oral antibiotic therapy (using rifampicin and clarithromycin). The use of an oral antibiotic regimen will ensure that more people have access to treatment, and thereby allow the roadmap's second target to be reached: curing 70% of cases in endemic countries by 2020 (*20*).

REFERENCES

1   *Buruli ulcer* (Mycobacterium ulcerans *infection*). Geneva, World Health Organization, 2012 (Fact sheet No. 199) (http://who.int/mediacentre/factsheets/fs199/en/index.html; accessed November 2012).

2   Ngoa UA et al. Buruli ulcer in Gabon, 2001–2010. *Emerging Infectious Diseases*, 2012, 18:1206–1207.

3   Agbenorku P et al. Buruli-ulcer induced disability in Ghana: a study at Apromase in the Ashanti Region. *Plastic Surgery International*, 2012, 2012:752749 (doi:10.1155/2012/752749).

4   Boyd SC et al. Epidemiology, clinical features and diagnosis of *Mycobacterium ulcerans* in an Australian population. *Medical Journal of Australia*, 2012, 196:341–344.

5   *Abstracts of the annual meeting on Buruli ulcer: 14–17 March 2005*. Geneva, World Health Organization, 2006 (http://www.who.int/buruli/information/publications/REPORT_2005_FINAL.pdf; accessed November 2012).

6   Buruli ulcer disease. *Mycobacterium ulcerans* infection: an overview of reported cases globally. *Weekly Epidemiological Record*, 2004, 79:194–199.

7   Amofah G et al. Buruli ulcer in Ghana: results of a national case search. *Emerging Infectious Diseases*, 2002, 8:167–170.

8   Yotsu RR et al. Buruli ulcer and current situation in Japan: a new emerging cutaneous *Mycobacterium* infection. *Journal of Dermatology*, 2012, 37:587–593.

9   *Buruli ulcer: number of new cases reported*. WHO Global Health Observatory Data Repository (http://apps.who.int/gho/data).

10 Asiedu K, Etuaful S. Socioeconomic implications of Buruli ulcer in Ghana: a three-year review. *American Journal of Tropical Medicine and Hygiene*, 1998, 59:1015–1022.

11 VanderWerf TS et al. *Mycobacterium ulcerans* infection. *Lancet*, 1999, 354:1013–1018.

12 Toll A. Aggressive multifocal Buruli ulcer with associated osteomyelitis in an HIV-positive patient. *Clinical and Experimental Dermatology*, 2005, 30:649–651.

13 Kibadi D et al. Buruli ulcer lesions in HIV-positive patient. *Emerging Infectious Diseases*, 2010, 16:738–739.

14 *Economic burden of Buruli ulcer on households in the Central and Ashanti regions of Ghana. Report of the 7th WHO Advisory Group Meeting on Buruli ulcer, 8–11 March 2004*. Geneva, World Health Organization, 2004 (WHO/CDS/CPE/GBUI/2004.9).

15 Drummond C, Butler JRG. *Mycobacterium ulcerans* treatment costs, self-reported data, Australia. *Emerging Infectious Diseases*, 2004, 10:1038–1043.

16 Peeters Grietens K et al. "It is me who endures but my family that suffers": social isolation as a consequence of the household cost burden of Buruli ulcer free of charge hospital treatment. *PLoS Neglected Tropical Diseases*, 2008, 2:e321 (doi:10.1371/journal.pntd.0000321).

17 *Cotonou declaration on Buruli ulcer*. Geneva, World Health Organization, 2009.

18 *Treatment of* Mycobacterium ulcerans *disease (Buruli ulcer): guidance for health workers*. Geneva, World Health Organization, 2012 (WHO/HTM/NTD/IDM/2012.1).

19 Chauty A et al. Promising clinical efficacy of streptomycin-rifampin combination for treatment of Buruli ulcer (*Mycobacterium ulcerans* disease). *Antimicrobial Agents and Chemotherapy*, 2007, 51:4029–4035.

20 *Accelerating work to overcome the global impact of neglected tropical diseases: a roadmap for implementation*. Geneva, World Health Organization, 2012 (WHO/HTM/NTD/2012.1).

3.5 ENDEMIC TREPONEMATOSES

Introduction

Endemic treponematoses, comprising yaws, endemic syphilis (bejel) and pinta, result from infection with bacteria of the genus *Treponema*. Yaws is the commonest of the three diseases. Mass treatment campaigns led by WHO and UNICEF between 1952 and 1964 reduced the prevalences of treponematoses from 50 million to 2.5 million (*1*). Progress was not sustained, however, and treponematoses resurged in the 1970s. Yaws, which is not a fatal disease, most frequently infects children, and cases peak among those aged 2–10 years (*2*). Children younger than 15 years account for 75% of new cases. For pinta, the age range is 10–30 years. Yaws affects boys more often than girls; there is no difference between males and females in the numbers affected by endemic syphilis and pinta.

Distribution

The global extent of endemic treponematoses is not known accurately. The most recent data, based on routine surveillance from some countries, are shown in *Fig. 3.5.1* and *Table 3.5.1*. Since reporting yaws is not mandatory, these figures provide no more than an indication of the distribution of the disease (*3*).

Fig. 3.5.1 Global distribution of endemic treponematoses, 2008–2011

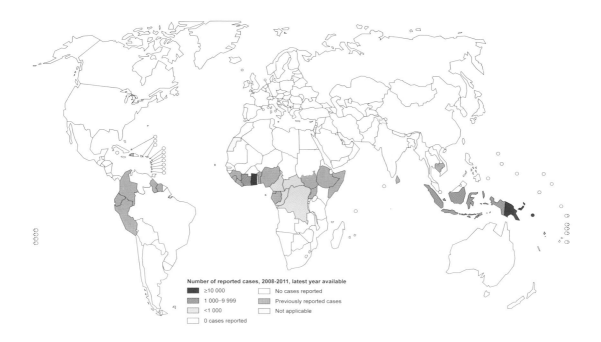

Number of reported cases, 2008-2011, latest year available

- ≥10 000
- 1 000–9 999
- <1 000
- 0 cases reported
- No cases reported
- Previously reported cases
- Not applicable

DISEASES

Table 3.5.1 Countries reporting data on yaws, by WHO region, 2008–2011 (3, 4)

WHO region, country (and year) of report	Number of cases
African	
Benin[a]	No data available
Cameroon (2010)	789
Central African Republic (2008)	243
Congo (2010)	167
Côte d'Ivoire (2010)	3 704
Democratic Republic of the Congo (2009)	383
Ghana (2010)	20 525
Togo (2010)	15
Americas[b]	–
South-East Asia	
India[c]	0
Indonesia (2011)	5 319
Timor-Leste[a]	No data available
Western Pacific	
Papua New Guinea (2011)	34 628
Solomon Islands (2010)	20 635
Vanuatu (2010)	1 574

[a] Country known to be endemic.
[b] No data on yaws are available for the Region of the Americas. A report published in 2003 (Anselmi M et al. Community participation eliminates yaws in Ecuador. *Tropical Medicine and International Health,* 8:634–638) declared that yaws had been eliminated in Ecuador. A review paper published in 1977 (Hopkins DR. Yaws in the Americas 1950–1975. *Journal of Infectious Diseases,* 136:548–554) indicated that yaws and pinta were no longer public-health problems in the region.
[c] India interrupted transmission in 2004 and declared elimination in 2006. Since 2004, no new cases have been reported.

Impact

Ulcers may become infected, and this may lead to severe secondary bacterial infection, including tetanus. Long-term complications of yaws (arising 5 or more years after the onset of infection) occur in 10% of untreated cases, causing disfigurement of the face and legs. Children aged 2–14 years are most badly affected, and serve as the main reservoir of infection for yaws and endemic syphilis. In late stages, yaws can cause disfiguring and crippling disabilities and deformities that prevent children from going to school and adults from physical labour. Thus there are social, economic, humanitarian and ethical considerations that justify the intensification of efforts to eradicate yaws.

Strategy (roadmap targets and milestones)

Effective and inexpensive treatment is available for treponematoses. Treatment can now be accomplished with a single oral dose of azithromycin or, in instances where azithromycin is not available or appropriate, a single injection of long-acting benzathine benzylpenicillin (*3,4,5,6*). Consequently, yaws has been targeted for eradication by 2020.

In March 2012, WHO convened a meeting of experts to develop a strategy for eradicating yaws in view of the new finding on azithromycin. The meeting recommended two new treatment policies to replace those developed in the 1950s (*6*). These new policies are: (i) to deliver mass treatment to an entire endemic community irrespective of the number of active clinical cases and to follow this with regular surveillance until clinical cases are no longer identified; and (ii) to deliver targeted treatment to all active clinical cases and their contacts (household, school, and playmates), an approach that requires support from existing health-care services.

When oral azithromycin is used for mass treatment, transmission can be interrupted within 6 months, as was shown in the Nsukka district of Nigeria (*7*). Accordingly, WHO plans to initiate large-scale treatment in endemic areas in Cameroon, Ghana, Indonesia, Papua New Guinea, the Solomon Islands and Vanuatu (*3*). The experience gained from these pilot interventions will be used to guide the timeline for global eradication (*Table 3.5.2*).

Table 3.5.2 Targets and milestones for eradicating yaws

Year	Milestone					
2012	Status of endemic countries in South-East Asia and Western Pacific regions completed					
2013	Assessment of endemic countries completed in the African Region	New strategy for yaws eradication incorporated into national policies in all regions	Criteria for verifying interruption of transmission developed	Mechanisms for monitoring and evaluation established	Agreements for donations of azithromycin finalized to ensure success of eradication efforts	International advisory body and international verification team established
2015	50% of endemic countries report zero cases					
2017	100% of endemic countries have report zero cases					
2020	Interruption of transmission verified in all countries					

DISEASES

REFERENCES

1. Perine PL et al. *Handbook of endemic treponematoses: yaws, endemic syphilis and pinta*. Geneva, World Health Organization, 1984.

2. Meheus AZ, Narain JP, Asiedu KB. Endemic treponematoses. In: Cohen J, Powderly SM, Opal WG, eds. *Infectious diseases*, 3rd ed. London, Mosby Elsevier, 2010:1106–1109.

3. Eradication of yaws – the Morges strategy. *Weekly Epidemiological Record*, 2012, 87:189–194.

4. Mitjà O et al. Single-dose azithromycin versus benzathine benzylpenicillin for treatment of yaws in children in Papua New Guinea: an open-label, non-inferiority, randomized trial. *Lancet*, 2012, 379:342–347.

5. Mitjà O et al. New treatment schemes for yaws: the path toward eradication. *Clinical Infectious Diseases*, 2012 (doi:10.1093/cid/cis444).

6. *Summary report of a consultation on the eradication of yaws: 5–7 March 2012, Morges, Switzerland.* Geneva, World Health Organization, 2012 (WHO/HTM/NTD/IDM/2012.2).

7. Yaws eradication campaign in Nsukka division, eastern Nigeria – a preliminary review. *Bulletin of the World Health Organization*, 1956, 15:911–935.

3.6   LEPROSY

Introduction

Leprosy is a complex disease caused by infection with *Mycobacterium leprae*. The course and pathology of the disease depend on the response of the person's immune system to the infection. Most control programmes use clinical criteria for classifying and deciding on the appropriate treatment regimen for individual patients, particularly when skin-smear services are unavailable. The clinical system of classification uses the number of skin lesions and nerves involved to group patients into categories of either multibacillary leprosy or paucibacillary leprosy.

The integration of primary leprosy-control services with primary health-care services, and effective collaborations, have led to a considerable reduction in the burden of leprosy. Nevertheless, new cases occur in endemic countries, and areas with a high burden of the disease can exist against a low-burden background.

Distribution

By the beginning of 2012, 106 countries had submitted reports on leprosy to WHO (*1*): 29 from the African Region, 28 from the Region of the Americas, 11 from the South-East Asia Region, 22 from the Eastern Mediterranean Region and 16 from the Western Pacific Region. Mid-year population data for 2011 published by the Population Division of the United Nations Department of Economic and Social Affairs have been used to calculate rates (*2*). Most Member States in the European Region have not reported new cases recently, although several detect a few cases annually. WHO's Global Leprosy Programme has contacted the Member States in the European Region that reported only a few cases, and preliminary data for 2011 have been obtained. Once validated, these data will be published in the *Weekly Epidemiological Record*. The global situation is summarized in *Fig. 3.6.1*.

The regional distribution of leprosy at the beginning of 2012 is shown in *Table 3.6.1*. The total number of new cases detected in 2011 and reported by 106 countries was 224 355. Globally, the number of new cases of leprosy reported during the first quarter of 2012 was 181 941.

Fig. 3.6.1 New case-detection rates for leprosy, reported to WHO by January 2012

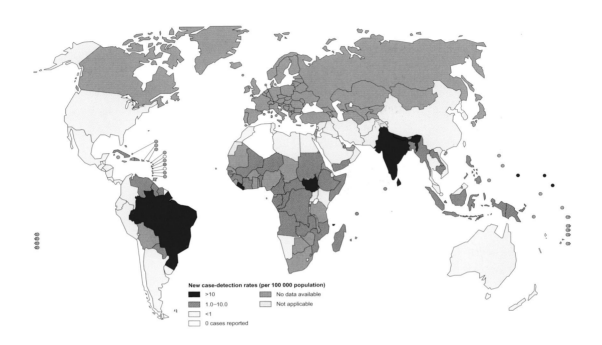

Table 3.6.1 Number of cases of leprosy (registered prevalence) in 106 countries or territories, by WHO region, 2011 and end of first quarter of 2012

WHO region[a]	No. of cases registered (prevalence rate),[b] first quarter 2012		No. of new cases detected (case-detection rate),[c] 2011	
African	15 006	(0.37)	17 953	(3.2)
Americas	34 801	(0.40)	36 832	(4.2)
South-East Asia	117 147	(0.64)	160 132	(8.8)
Eastern Mediterranean	7 368	(0.12)	4 346	(0.7)
Western Pacific	7 619	(0.05)	5 092	(0.3)
Total	181 941	(0.34)	224 355	(4.1)

[a] Reports from the European Region are not included.
[b] The prevalence rate is the number of cases/10 000 population.
[c] The case-detection rate is the number of cases/100 000 population.

The number of new cases detected annually continues to increase in all regions, except in the African and the Americas regions (*Table 3.6.2*). The apparent decline in the African Region reflects the low number of reports submitted, particularly from Member States that had previously reported high numbers of new cases.

Table 3.6.2 Number of new cases of leprosy, by WHO region, 2004–2011

WHO region[a]	No. of new cases detected							
	2004	2005	2006	2007	2008	2009	2010	2011
African	46 918	45 179	34 480	34 468	29 814	28 935	25 345	17 953
Americas	52 662	41 952	47 612	42 135	41 891	40 474	37 740	36 832
South-East Asia	298 603	201 635	174 118	171 576	167 505	166 115	156 254	160 132
Eastern Mediterranean	3 392	3 133	3 261	4 091	3 938	4 029	4 080	4 346
Western Pacific	6 216	7 137	6 190	5 863	5 859	5 243	5 055	5 092
Total	407 791	299 036	265 661	258 133	249 007	244 796	228 474	224 355

[a] Reports from the European Region are not included.

Impact

The number of new cases detected during 2011 in the 13 countries that previously reported 1000 or more new cases and the number of new cases detected annually since 2004 in countries reporting 1000 or more new cases in 2010 are shown in *Table 3.6.3*. The 19 countries that reported 1000 or more new cases during 2004–2011 account for 94% of the new cases detected worldwide in 2011. Of these countries, eight are in the African Region; however, Nigeria and the United Republic of Tanzania did not report data for 2011, thereby contributing to the decline in the data from the region.

DISEASES

Table 3.6.3 Number of new cases of leprosy detected in countries previously reporting ≥1000 new cases, 2011, and number of new cases detected annually 2004–2010

Country	No. of new cases detected							
	2004	2005	2006	2007	2008	2009	2010	2011
Angola	2 109	1 877	1 078	1 269	1 184	937	1 076	508
Bangladesh	8 242	7 882	6 280	5 357	5 249	5 239	3 848	3 970
Brazil	49 384	38 410	44 436	39 125	38 914	37 610	34 894	33 955
China	1 499	1 658	1 506	1 526	1 614	1 597	1 324	1 144
Democratic Republic of the Congo	11 781	10 369	8 257	8 820	6 114	5 062	5 049	3 949
India	260 063	169 709	139 252	137 685	134 184	133 717	126 800	127 295
Ethiopia	4 787	4 698	4 092	4 187	4 170	4 417	4 430	5 280
Indonesia	16 549	19 695	17 682	17 723	17 441	17 260	17 012	20 023
Madagascar	3 710	2 709	1 536	1 644	1 763	1 572	1 520	1 577
Mozambique	4 266	5 371	3 637	2 510	1 313	1 191	1 207	1 097
Myanmar	3 748	3 571	3 721	3 637	3 365	3 147	2 936	3 082
Nepal	6 958	6 150	4 235	4 436	4 708	4 394	3 118	3 184
Nigeria	5 276	5 024	3 544	4 665	4 899	4 219	3 913	NA
Philippines	2 254	3 130	2 517	2 514	2 373	1 795	2 041	1 818
Sri Lanka	1 995	1 924	1 993	2 024	1 979	1 875	2 027	2 178
Sudan	722	720	884	1 706[a]	1 901[a]	2 100[a]	2 394[a]	706
South Sudan	–	–	–	–	–	–	–	1 799
United Republic of Tanzania	5 190	4 237	3 450	3 105	3 276	2 654	2 349	NA
Total (%)	388 533 (95)	287 134 (96)	248 100 (93)	241 933 (94)	234 447 (94)	228 786 (93)	215 938 (95)	211 565 (94)
Global total	407 791	299 036	265 661	258 133	249 007	244 796	228 474	224 355

[a] Includes data from an area that is now South Sudan.
NA = not available

Data on multibacillary leprosy, the proportion of cases among women and children, and those with grade-2 disabilities are shown in *Table 3.6.4*. The proportion of cases with multibacillary leprosy among new leprosy cases in the African Region ranged from 89.52% in Kenya to 34.86% in the Comoros; in the Region of the Americas the proportion ranged from 84.12% in Argentina to 33.93% in Ecuador; in the South-East Asia Region it ranged from 80.40% in Indonesia to 44.98% in Sri Lanka; in the Eastern Mediterranean Region it ranged from 89.52% in Egypt to 52.17% in Yemen; in the Western Pacific Region the range was from 91.20% in the Philippines to 35.14% in Kiribati.

DISEASES

Table 3.6.4 Countries with highest and lowest proportions of newly detected cases of leprosy in countries reporting ≥100 new cases, by type of case and WHO region, 2011

WHO region[a]	% cases of multibacillary leprosy among new cases	% of females among new cases of leprosy	% of children among new cases of leprosy	% of new leprosy cases with grade-2 disabilities
African	Kenya, 89.52 Comoros, 34.86	Liberia, 57.55 Madagascar, 20.86	Comoros, 38.25 Burundi, 1.12	Madagascar, 21.64 Cameroon, 4.89
Americas	Argentina, 84.12 Ecuador, 33.93	Dominican Republic, 46.75 Paraguay, 31.20	Dominican Republic, 12.34 Argentina, 0.59	Colombia, 9.45 Mexico, 5.58
South-East Asia	Indonesia, 80.40 Sri Lanka, 44.98	Indonesia, 39.79 Nepal, 28.55	Indonesia, 12.25 Thailand, 6.43	Myanmar, 15.02 India, 3.01
Eastern Mediterranean	Egypt, 89.52 Yemen, 52.17	Somalia, 49.02 Pakistan, 40.56	South Sudan, 10.78 Sudan, 2.27	Somalia, 24.31 Egypt, 6.47
Western Pacific	Philippines, 91.20 Kiribati, 35.14	Marshall Islands, 43.88 Malaysia, 28.24	Marshall Islands, 39.66 China, 2.53	China, 27.01 Kiribati and the Marshall Islands, 0.0

[a] Reports from the European Region are not included.

The proportion of females among newly detected cases of leprosy ranged in the African Region from 57.55% in Liberia to 20.86% in Madagascar; in the Region of the Americas the range was from 46.75% in the Dominican Republic to 31.20% in Paraguay; in the South-East Asia Region the range was from 39.79% in Indonesia to 28.55% in Nepal; in the Eastern Mediterranean Region the range was from 49.02% in Somalia to 40.56% in Pakistan; and in the Western Pacific Region it was from 43.88% in the Marshall Islands to 28.24% in Malaysia.

The proportion of children among new cases of leprosy in the African Region ranged from 38.25% in the Comoros to 1.12% in Burundi; in the Region of the Americas it ranged from 12.34% in the Dominican Republic to 0.59% in Argentina; in the South-East Asia Region it ranged from 12.25% in Indonesia to 6.43% in Thailand; in the Eastern Mediterranean Region it ranged from 10.78% in South Sudan to 2.27% in Sudan; and in the Western Pacific Region the range was from 39.66% in the Marshall Islands to 2.53% in China.

DISEASES

The proportion of new cases with grade-2 disabilities (that is, visible disabilities) ranged in the African Region from 4.89% in Cameroon to 21.64% in Madagascar; in the Region of the Americas from 9.45% in Colombia to 5.58% in Mexico; in the South-East Asia Region from 15.02% in Myanmar to 3.01% in India; in the Eastern Mediterranean Region from 24.31% in Somalia to 6.47% in Egypt; and in the Western Pacific Region from 27.01% in China to 0% reported by the Marshall Islands and Kiribati.

The trends from 2005 to 2011 for new cases with grade-2 disabilities and rates/100 000 population are shown in *Table 3.6.5*. In 2011, the global rate of new cases with grade-2 disabilities was 0.23. Also during 2011, a total of 12 225 new cases with grade-2 disabilities was detected, a slight reduction compared with 2010 (13 275 cases). In 2011, the rate of new cases with grade-2 disabilities ranged from 0.03 in the Western Pacific Region to 0.39 in the South-East Asia Region.

Table 3.6.5 Number of cases of leprosy (rate/100 000 of population) with grade-2 disabilities detected among new leprosy cases, by WHO region, 2005–2011

WHO region[a]	Year						
	2004	2005	2006	2007	2008	2009	2010
African	4 562 (0.62)	3 244 (0.46)	3 570 (0.51)	3 458(0.51)	3 146 (0.41)	2 685 (0.40)	1 446 (0.36)
Americas	2 107 (0.25)	2 302 (0.27)	3 431 (0.42)	2 512 (0.29)	2 645 (0.30)	2 423 (0.27)	2 382 (0.27)
South-East Asia	6 209 (0.37)	5 791 (0.35)	6 332 (0.37)	6 891 (0.39)	7 286 (0.41)	6 912 (0.39)	7 095 (0.39)
Eastern Mediterranean	335 (0.07)	384 (0.08)	466 (0.10)	687 (0.14)	608 (0.11)	729 (0.12)	753 (0.12)
Western Pacific	673 (0.04)	671 (0.04)	604 (0.03)	592 (0.03)	635 (0.04)	526 (0.03)	549 (0.03)
Total	13 886 (0.25)	12 392 (0.23)	14 403 (0.26)	14 140 (0.25)	14 320 (0.25)	13 275 (0.23)	12 225 (0.23)

[a] Reports from the European Region are not included.

Trends in the number of relapsed cases reported globally from 2004 to 2011 are shown in *Table 3.6.6*. The number of relapsed cases reported in 2011 (2921) exceeded that reported in 2010 (2113).

DISEASES

Table 3.6.6 Number of relapsed cases of leprosy reported worldwide, 2004–2011

Year	No. of countries reporting	No. of relapsed cases
2004	40	2 439
2005	44	2 783
2006	41	2 270
2007	43	2 466
2008	49	2 985
2009	122	3 120
2010	117	2 113
2011	96	2 921

Strategy (roadmap targets and milestones)

Plans to eliminate leprosy worldwide as a public-health problem by 2020 have been prepared, and their implementation is progressing. The *Enhanced global strategy for further reducing the disease burden due to leprosy (plan period: 2011–2015)* (*3*) is being implemented by national programmes in endemic countries. The strategy aims to reduce the global rate of new cases with grade-2 disabilities per 1 million population by at least 35% by the end of 2015; the baseline for comparison is the end of 2010. This approach underlines the importance of detecting cases early, providing multidrug therapy early, and ensuring a high standard of care in a setting of integrated services. Whether the elimination target is achieved depends on the following five components of the strategy:

1. Implementing WHO's strategy in all endemic countries by 2013;

2. Reducing the burden of disease at subnational levels by 2015 (at least 50% of new cases and at least 35% of new cases with disabilities). This will be achieved by (i) implementing advocacy and awareness campaigns that will be followed by intensified leprosy detection and treatment at the local level in countries that report more than 1 000 new cases annually, and (ii) improving the specificity of diagnosis by using clinical or other investigations;

3. Strengthening capacity to intensify and sustain leprosy-control activities by (i) establishing or strengthening institutions that conduct regular courses about leprosy diagnosis and treatment and organizing training workshops at the subnational level, and (ii) organizing annual intercountry and regional meetings of national programme managers to review programmes' performance and share experiences;

4. Reducing stigma and discrimination. Countries have agreed to implement the principles of the United Nations resolution on the elimination of stigma and discrimination against persons affected by leprosy and their families (*4*). This will be achieved by encouraging collaboration among relevant ministries, including social services, education and justice, as well as with other partners to expand welfare and development programmes for people affected by leprosy, by engaging in regular advocacy and encouraging the goodwill ambassador for leprosy elimination to regularly visit affected countries;

5. Intensifying research by investing in the development of diagnostics and treatment, and working to prevent neuritis. Additionally, coordinating operational research should help to increase early diagnosis and the quality of leprosy services.

REFERENCES

[1] Global leprosy situation, 2012. *Weekly Epidemiological Record*, 2012, 87:317–328.

[2] *World population prospects: the 2006 revision*, vol. 1. New York, United Nations, 2007:578–586.

[3] *Enhanced global strategy for further reducing the disease burden due to leprosy (plan period: 2011–2015)*. New Delhi, World Health Organization, Regional Office for South-East Asia, 2009 (SEA-GLP-2009.3).

[4] *Resolution 8/13: elimination of discrimination against persons affected by leprosy and their family members*. Geneva, United Nations Human Rights Council, 2008.

3.7   CHAGAS DISEASE

Introduction

Chagas disease is caused by infection with the protozoa *Trypanosoma cruzi*. Transmission to humans usually occurs through (i) contact with faeces of vector insects (triatomine bugs), including the ingestion of contaminated food, (ii) transfusion of infected blood, (iii) congenital transmission, (iv) organ transplantation or (v) laboratory accidents (*1*).

Distribution

About 7 million to 8 million people worldwide are estimated to be infected with *T. cruzi*, mostly in the endemic areas of 21 Latin American countries: Argentina, Belize, the Bolivarian Republic of Venezuela, Brazil, Chile, Colombia, Costa Rica, Ecuador, El Salvador, French Guyana, Guatemala, Guyana, Honduras, Mexico, Nicaragua, Panama, Paraguay, Peru, the Plurinational State of Bolivia, Suriname and Uruguay (*2*) (*Fig. 3.7.1*).

Fig. 3.7.1 Global distribution of cases of Chagas disease, based on official estimates, 2006–2010

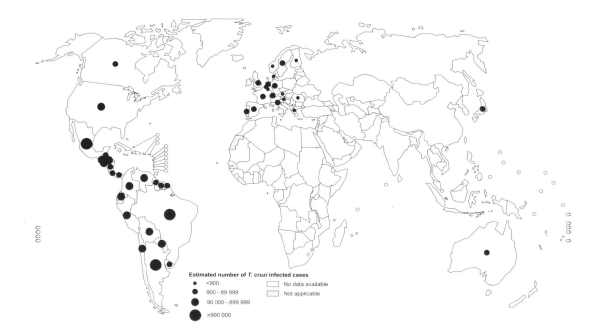

Estimated number of *T. cruzi* infected cases

- • <900
- • 900 – 89 999
- • 90 000 – 899 999
- • ≥900 000

No data available
Not applicable

The presence of Chagas disease outside Latin America mainly results from population mobility, predominantly migration (*3*), but may also occur when travellers to Latin America return to their home countries (*4*).

Impact

The changing epidemiological pattern of *T. cruzi* combined with the spread of HIV has led to coinfection and comorbidity. These two chronic infections met in the 1980s following population movement and urbanization (*5*). Despite coinfections often being underdiagnosed, several countries – including Argentina, the Bolivarian Republic of Venezuela, Brazil, Chile, Colombia, Italy, Mexico, Paraguay, Spain, the United States of America and Uruguay – have reported cases of coinfection, with the highest prevalences occurring in the south of the Region of the Americas and southern Europe (*Fig. 3.7.2*).

The cost of treatment for Chagas disease remains substantial. In Colombia alone, the annual cost of medical care for all patients with the disease has been estimated to be about US$ 267 million. Spraying insecticide to control vectors would cost nearly US$ 5 million annually (*6*).

Fig. 3.7.2 Global distribution of cases diagnosed and published with *Trypanosoma cruzi* and HIV coinfection, 2006–2010

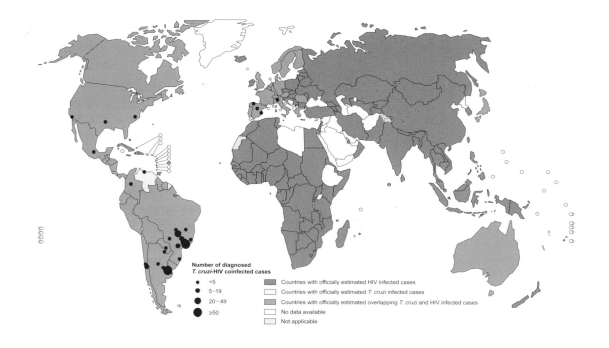

Strategy (roadmap targets and milestones)

WHO's targets for the control and elimination of Chagas disease are based on two pillars: interrupting transmission and providing care for patients. Efforts to reduce transmission include: interrupting intradomiciliary vectorial transmission and reducing the risk of oral transmission (in Latin America); and interrupting transmission acquired through blood transfusions and organ transplantation (in Latin America, Europe and the Western Pacific).

The two-pillar strategy is supported by data from active information and surveillance systems at the country, regional and global levels that detect active transmission routes, infected and ill people, congenital cases and degree of effective patient care. Vector control –mainly spraying homes with insecticides that leave residues (residual insecticides) – also involves making improvements to dwellings, improving hygiene in houses to prevent insect infestation. Key measures to control vector-related transmission also include improving sanitation, implementing personal control measures (such as using bednets) and practising good hygiene when preparing, transporting, storing and consuming food. Screening blood from donors and organ donors are also fundamental methods to interrupt transmission.

REFERENCES

[1] *Working to overcome the global impact of neglected tropical diseases: first WHO report on neglected tropical diseases.* Geneva, World Health Organization, 2010 (WHO/HTM/NTD/2010.1).

[2] *Quantitative estimation of Chagas disease in the Americas.* Montevideo, Pan American Health Organization, 2006 (OPS/HDM/CD/425-06).

[3] Coura JR, Vinas PA. Chagas disease: a new worldwide challenge. *Nature*, 2010, 465(Suppl.):S6–S7.

[4] Sztajzel et al. Chagas' disease may also be encountered in Europe. *European Heart Journal*, 1996, 17:1289–1291.

[5] Livramento JA, Machado LR, Spina França A. Anormalidades do líquido cefalorraqueano em 170 casos de AIDS [Cephalorachidian fluid abnormalities in 170 AIDS cases]. *Arquivos de Neuro-Psiquiatria*, 1989, 47: 326–331.

[6] Castillo-Riquelme M et al. The costs of preventing and treating Chagas disease in Colombia. *PLoS Neglected Tropical Diseases*, 2008, 2:e336.

3.8   HUMAN AFRICAN TRYPANOSOMIASIS (SLEEPING SICKNESS)

Introduction

Human African trypanosomiasis, or sleeping sickness, is caused by infection with protozoan parasites belonging to the genus *Trypanosoma*. The disease is vector-borne; parasites enter the body through the bites of tsetse flies (*Glossina* spp.). Without prompt diagnosis and treatment, the disease is usually fatal: the parasites multiply in the body, cross the blood–brain barrier and invade the central nervous system.

Distribution

Since 2009, the number of new cases reported annually has been fewer than 10 000 for the first time in 50 years, with 9875 new cases in 2009, 7139 in 2010 and 6743 in 2011. This trend represents a decrease of 72% during the past 10 years. The number of cases reported annually is considered to be a fraction of the real number of infected individuals. According to the latest 2011 estimates (*1*), the incidence could be around 20 000 cases a year.

The chronic form of human African trypanosomiasis, caused by infection with *Trypanosoma brucei gambiense*, is endemic in 24 countries, and represents 98% of reported cases (*Fig. 3.8.1*). During 2009, 2010 and 2011, Benin, Burkina Faso, Ghana, Mali and Togo continued reporting zero cases. No cases have been reported during the past 30 years in the Gambia, Guinea-Bissau, Liberia, Niger, Senegal and Sierra Leone despite no specific control activities having been conducted; field assessment is needed to verify the epidemiological status in these countries. Cameroon, the Congo, Côte d'Ivoire, Equatorial Guinea, Gabon, Guinea, Nigeria and Uganda reported fewer than 100 new cases annually; Angola, the Central African Republic, Chad and South Sudan reported between 100 and 1000 new cases annually. The Democratic Republic of the Congo is the only country that has reported more than 1000 new cases annually, and it accounts for 84% of the cases reported in 2011. The largest proportion of reported cases of sleeping sickness (96.5%) occur in WHO's African Region; the Eastern Mediterranean Region accounts for the remaining 3.5%.

The acute form of human African trypanosomiasis, caused by infection with *Trypanosoma brucei rhodesiense*, is endemic in 13 countries, and represents 2% of all cases of the disease reported during 2009–2011 (*Fig. 3.8.2*). Botswana, Namibia and Swaziland, considered to be endemic, have not reported any cases in the past 20 years; in these countries, the vector appears to be no longer present. Data are not

Fig. 3.8.1 Global distribution of human African trypanosomiasis (caused by *Trypanosoma brucei gambiense*), 2011

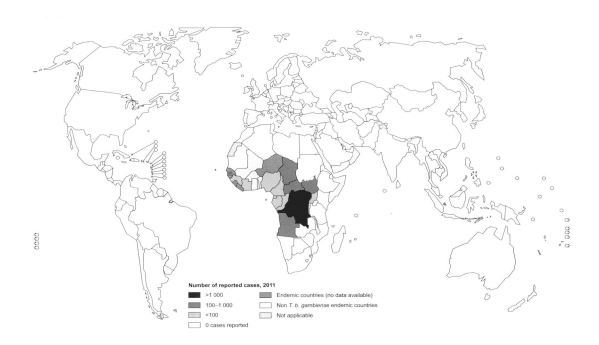

Fig. 3.8.2 Global distribution of human African trypanosomiasis (caused by *Trypanosoma brucei rhodesiense*), 2011

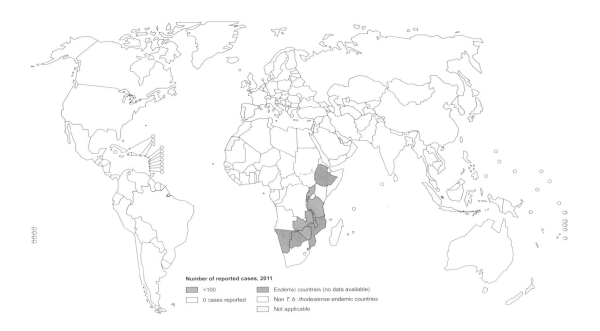

DISEASES

available from Burundi, Ethiopia, Mozambique and Rwanda, and field studies are needed to clarify the epidemiological status. Kenya and Zimbabwe have reported sporadic cases; Malawi, the United Republic of Tanzania and Zambia have reported fewer than 100 new cases annually; Uganda has reported between 100 and less than 200 new cases annually. More detailed information about the distribution of the disease is available in WHO's atlas of human African trypanosomiasis (*2*).

Impact

Human African trypanosomiasis affects impoverished rural areas of sub-Saharan Africa, where it coexists with animal trypanosomiasis; the presence of both forms of the disease impedes development in these communities and traps people in a cycle of poverty.

Approximately 70 million people distributed over an area of 1.55 million km^2 are at risk (*3*). Advances in controlling the disease made during the past decade have achieved an important decrease in its burden, but control and research efforts must continue and be based on sustainable public-health objectives, not only on the actual burden of the disease. The decline in the numbers of cases is shown in *Fig. 3.8.3*; this decline reflects a drop in the burden of disease.

Fig. 3.8.3 Global number of new cases of human African trypanosomiasis reported to WHO, 1990–2011

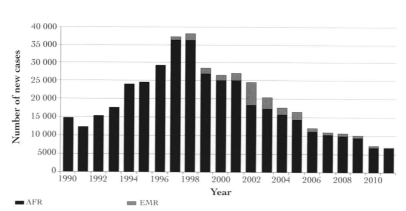

AFR – African Region / EMR–Eastern Mediterranean Region

Strategy (roadmap targets and milestones)

Reaching the roadmap's targets for eliminating human African trypanosomiasis depends on increasing access to early, accurate diagnosis; delivering safer and effective treatment; and continuing surveillance. Crucial stages for reaching the roadmap's targets are shown in *Table 3.8.1*.

Table 3.8.1 Indicators and milestones in eliminating human African trypanosomiasis

Indicators and milestones for disease elimination	Year								
	2012	2013	2014	2015	2016	2017	2018	2019	2020
Define elimination criteria	√								
Establish Expert Committee on control and surveillance		√							
Provide annual update of number of people at risk covered by control activities	√	√	√	√	√	√	√	√	√
Provide biennial update of disease distribution	√		√		√		√		√
Provide biennial update of number of people at risk	√		√		√		√		√
Convene biennial follow-up meetings with affected countries			√		√		√		√
Follow up with partners annually	√	√	√	√	√	√	√	√	√
Targets for global number of cases reported annually	6000	5500	5000	4500	4000	3500	3000	2500	>2000
Proportion of foci where elimination validated (<1 case/10 000 population)				10%	30%	40%	60%	80%	>90%

Since 2007, efforts have been made to switch to melarsoprol-free treatments by supplying national control programmes with a standardized kit of materials needed to administer combined nifurtimox–eflornithine therapy to treat second-stage infection with *T. b. gambiense*. Kits may be obtained free from WHO together with training organized by WHO for health-care workers. Sanofi and Bayer donate the medicines that are distributed by WHO in collaboration with Médecins Sans Frontières Logistique.

The use of toxic melarsoprol has declined markedly; by 2010, 88% of cases were treated with melarsoprol-free therapy. Because use of this new treatment was based on limited experience, a reinforced pharmacovigilance system was introduced in 2010. A total of 22 sentinel sites were set up in the Central African Republic, Chad, the Congo, Côte d'Ivoire, the Democratic Republic of the Congo, Equatorial Guinea, Guinea, South Sudan and Uganda. More than 1000 notifications of adverse effects have been received; these have helped to improve the routine use of the treatment and confirmed it as the best therapeutic option for treating second-stage sleeping sickness caused by *T. b. gambiense* (*4*). The distribution of medicines to treat cases of the disease diagnosed in travellers and migrants in countries where the disease is not endemic is supported by a separate surveillance system (*Fig. 3.8.4*) (*5*).

The use of melarsoprol-free treatment has imposed a financial burden on control programmes. In 2010, the average cost to treat one patient with second-stage gambiense sickness was US$ 440 compared with US$ 30 in 2001. This burden might render treatment unsustainable in the future; thus it is important that research continues to look for safe and effective medicines that are simpler to administer and cheaper than those currently available.

Fig. 3.8.4 Global distribution of cases of human African trypanosomiasis diagnosed in non-endemic countries and probable places of infection, 2000–2010

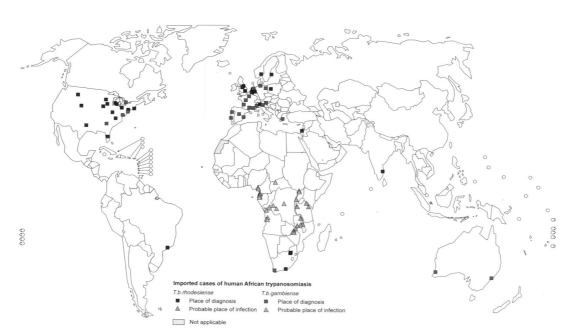

Imported cases of human African trypanosomiasis

T.b.rhodesiense
■ Place of diagnosis
△ Probable place of infection

T.b.gambiense
■ Place of diagnosis
△ Probable place of infection

☐ Not applicable

DISEASES

In 2009, WHO set up a specimen bank that is available to researchers to facilitate the development of new and affordable diagnostic tools. The bank contains samples of blood, serum, cerebrospinal fluid, saliva and urine from patients infected with both forms of the disease as well as samples from uninfected people from areas where the disease is endemic. Overall, samples have been obtained from 1798 participants in 6 countries (6).

As the number of new cases declines, new cost-effective approaches to integrate control and surveillance for the disease into health-care systems have been developed and are being tested in Benin and Togo. The control and surveillance system depends on the serological screening of selected patients who attend referral hospitals located in known foci of the disease. Positive samples are referred to WHO's collaborating centres for further analysis. This approach has been in place for 2 years, and there has been successful follow up and evaluation of it. The system will be extended to other endemic countries for further evaluation.

In collaboration with the FAO, under the framework of the Programme Against African Trypanosomiasis, WHO has strengthened surveillance by finalizing the atlas of human African trypanosomiasis (2). The atlas maps control activities and cases reported at village level during 2000–2009. The 36 endemic countries have completed their mapping, including 175 576 cases and 19 828 geographical sites (7). The atlas is a powerful tool that can help endemic countries prepare control strategies, carry out interventions, monitor their impact, and sustain progress through surveillance. Using the data in the atlas and population layers, a methodology has been developed to calculate at-risk populations (8).

REFERENCES

[1] Simarro PP et al. The Human African Trypanosomiasis Control and Surveillance Programme of the World Health Organization 2000–2009: the way forward. *PLoS Neglected Tropical Diseases*, 2011, 5:e1007 (doi:10.1371/journal.pntd.0001007).

[2] *Mapping the foci of human African trypanosomiasis*. Geneva, World Health Organization (http://www.who.int/trypanosomiasis_african/country/foci_AFRO/en/index.html; accessed November 2012).

[3] Simarro PP et al. Estimating and mapping the population at risk of sleeping sickness. *PLoS Neglected Tropical Diseases*, 2012, 6(10): e1859. (doi:10.1371/journal.pntd.0001859).

[4] Franco JR et al. Monitoring the use of nifurtimox-eflornithine combination therapy (NECT) in the treatment of second stage gambiense human African trypanosomiasis. *Reports and Research in Tropical Medicine*, 2012, 3:93–101.

[5] Simarro PP et al. Human African trypanosomiasis in non-endemic countries (2000–2010). *Journal of Travel Medicine*, 2012, 19:44–53.

DISEASES

6   Franco JR et al. The human African trypanosomiasis specimen biobank: a necessary tool to support research of new diagnostics. *PLoS Neglected Tropical Diseases*, 2012, 6(6):e1571 (doi:10.1371/journal.pntd.0001571).

7   Simarro PP et al. The atlas of human African trypanosomiasis: a contribution to global mapping of neglected tropical diseases. *International Journal of Health Geographics*, 2010, 9:57.

8   Simarro PP et al. Risk for human African trypanosomiasis, Central Africa, 2000–2009. *Emerging Infectious Diseases*, 2011, 17:2322–2324.

3.9   LEISHMANIASES

Introduction

The Leishmaniases are caused by protozoan parasites transmitted through the bites of infected female sandflies (*Phlebotomus, Psychodopygus, Lutzomyia*). Visceral Leishmaniasis, also known as kala-azar, is usually fatal within 2 years if left untreated. After treatment, visceral Leishmaniasis sometimes evolves into a cutaneous form known as post-kala-azar dermal Leishmaniasis, cases of which may serve as sources of infection for sandflies and so maintain transmission (*1*). Cutaneous Leishmaniasis is the most prevalent form, causing ulcers that heal spontaneously. The mucocutaneous form invades the mucous membranes of the upper respiratory tract, causing gross mutilation by destroying soft tissues in the nose, mouth and throat.

Distribution

The Leishmaniases are prevalent in 98 countries and 3 territories on 5 continents (*Fig. 3.9.1* and *Fig. 3.9.2*). Approximately 1.3 million new cases occur annually, of which 300 000 are visceral (90% of which occur in Bangladesh, Brazil, Ethiopia, India, Nepal, South Sudan and Sudan) and 1 million are cutaneous (occurring mainly in Afghanistan, Algeria, Brazil, Colombia, the Islamic Republic of Iran, Pakistan, Peru, Saudi Arabia, the Syrian Arab Republic and Tunisia) or mucocutaneous (mainly occurring in Brazil, Peru and the Plurinational State of Bolivia). Of the 1.3 million estimated cases, only about 600 000 are actually reported (*2*). The distribution of the Leishmaniases has expanded since 1993, and there has been an increase in the number of cases recorded (*3*). Since reporting is mandatory in only 33/98 affected countries, the true increase in cases remains unknown. The spread of the Leishmaniases is mostly caused by movement of populations that expose nonimmune people to transmission (*4*).

In South Sudan, an epidemic of visceral Leishmaniasis that lasted from 2009 to 2011 involved more than 25 000 cases and caused more than 700 deaths. The rapid response from WHO, Médecins Sans Frontières (MSF) and other partners in collaboration with the government, kept the mortality rate to below 5% compared with 35% in the epidemic that occurred during the 1990s.

Infection with HIV appears to increase susceptibility to visceral disease and affect its epidemiology. As of 2012, 35 disease-endemic countries have reported cases of coinfection with HIV and visceral Leishmaniasis. In places where there is insufficient access to antiretroviral therapy, the prevalence of visceral disease is rising. In northern Ethiopia, the rate of coinfected patients increased from 19% during 1998–1999 to 34% during 2006–2007 (*5*).

Fig. 3.9.1 Global distribution of visceral Leishmaniasis, 2010

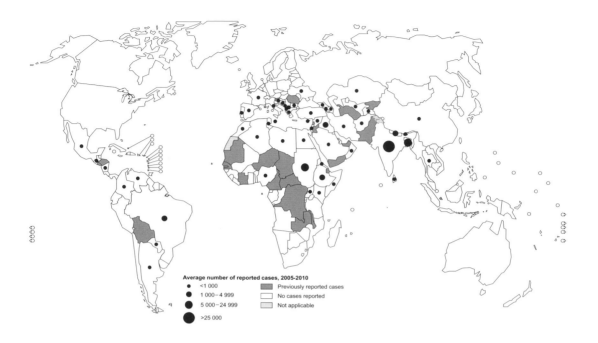

Fig. 3.9.2 Global distribution of cutaneous Leishmaniasis, 2010

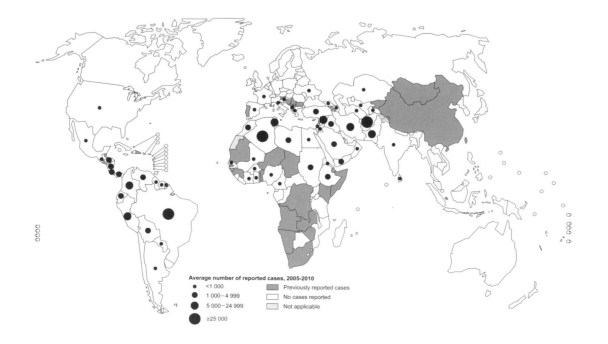

Epidemics of cutaneous Leishmaniasis have occurred in Afghanistan, where war and civil unrest have made its control difficult (6). In 2011, more than 30 000 cases of cutaneous disease were reported from all endemic areas in the country.

Impact

An estimated 20 000 to 40 000 people die from visceral Leishmaniasis annually (2). In East Africa, particularly in South Sudan and Sudan, epidemics of visceral disease, which has a high case-fatality rate, are frequent (7).

The health burden of cutaneous Leishmaniasis remains largely unknown, partly because those who are most affected live in remote areas and often do not seek medical attention. There is a psychosocial burden associated with the deformities and disfiguring scars that encourages patients to remain hidden. Cutaneous Leishmaniasis and mucocutaneous Leishmaniasis can lead to exclusion from society because of the mistaken belief that the disease is directly contagious. Mothers with cutaneous disease may refrain or be prohibited from touching their children; young women with scars are unable to marry (6); and the disease may provide the pretext for a husband to abandon a wife.

No comprehensive study has assessed the economic impact of the Leishmaniases. Most studies examine only the immediate impacts of the disease and the expenditures associated with treatment and patient care. These studies indicate that visceral Leishmaniasis has a negative effect on a significant portion of a household's income and contributes to a downward economic spiral (8,9).

Strategy (roadmap targets and milestones)

World Health Assembly resolution WHA60.13 on the control of Leishmaniasis was adopted in May 2007, and reinvigorated WHO's mandate to take a leading role in expanding control programmes (10). In March 2010, the WHO Expert Committee on the Control of the Leishmaniases met to develop guidelines for controlling these diseases (1). This meeting was followed by the publication of epidemiological information and an update on access to medicines (2). The epidemiological update identified gaps in the knowledge about the burden of the disease and incidence in most endemic countries, and drew attention to the need for developing robust surveillance systems. This work provides a secure base from which to reach the target of eliminating anthroponotic visceral Leishmaniasis on the Indian subcontinent by 2020. Crucial stages in achieving the roadmap's target are set out in *Table 3.9.1*.

In December 2011, WHO signed an agreement for the donation of 445 000 vials of liposomal amphotericin B to treat visceral Leishmaniasis. This medicine is effective,

DISEASES

Table 3.9.1 Targets and milestones for eliminating the Leishmaniases

Year	Milestone
2012	• Published post-kala-azar dermal Leishmaniasis case-management and control manual for health workers
	• Published guidelines for Eastern Mediterranean Region on case-management of cutaneous Leishmaniasis
	• Formulated 5-year strategic framework for controlling cutaneous Leishmaniasis in countries in the Eastern Mediterranean Region
	• Updated epidemiological information in endemic countries in Region of the Americas
	• Conducted epidemiological assessment in selected endemic countries in the European Region
2013	• Aim to implement national control programmes for visceral Leishmaniasis in 5 endemic African countries (Ethiopia, Kenya, South Sudan, Sudan and Uganda)
	• Aim to detect and treat >75% of visceral Leishmaniasis cases in endemic countries in East Africa
	• Update maps on cutaneous and visceral Leishmaniases at subdistrict level in endemic countries in the Region of the Americas
	• Adapt guidelines for control of cutaneous and visceral Leishmaniases in endemic countries in the European Region
2014	• Aim to detect and treat >90% of cases of visceral Leishmaniasis and post-kala-azar dermal Leishmaniasis in the South-East Asia Region
	• Complete district-level epidemiological assessment and mapping of cutaneous and visceral Leishmaniases in 50% of endemic African countries
	• Update treatment policy for coinfection with visceral Leishmaniasis and HIV using best available evidence
	• Enhance surveillance of cutaneous, mucocutaneous and visceral Leishmaniases in the Region of the Americas
2015	• Aim to detect and treat all cases of visceral Leishmaniasis and post-kala-azar dermal Leishmaniasis in the South-East Asia Region
	• Detect and manage >70% of cases of cutaneous Leishmaniasis in the Eastern Mediterranean Region
	• Detect and treat >90% of cases of cutaneous, mucocutaneous and visceral Leishmaniases in the Region of the Americas
	• Detect and treat >90% of cases of cutaneous and visceral Leishmaniases in all endemic countries in the European Region
	• Complete district-level mapping of cutaneous and visceral Leishmaniases in all endemic African countries
2016	• Detect and treat 90% of visceral Leishmaniasis cases in all endemic African countries
2017	• Aim to verify <1 case /10 000 population per year in 80% of endemic districts and subdistricts in the South-East Asia Region
2020	• Reduce the incidence of visceral Leishmaniasis to <1 case/10 000 population per year at district and subdistrict levels in the South-East Asia Region
	• Aim to detect and treat all cases in the African Region, Region of the Americas, the European Region and the Eastern Mediterranean Region
	• Detect and manage 85% of cutaneous Leishmaniasis cases in all endemic countries

has a good safety record and is the preferred treatment for visceral disease in the Indian subcontinent (*11*). The donation will provide treatment for more than 50 000 patients over 5 years in countries in South-East Asia and East Africa. Support provided by the British and Spanish governments and the pharmaceutical industry helps sustain national efforts in endemic countries to control and eliminate the disease. Where the infection affects only humans, transmission can be reduced by implementing a combination of active case-detection, early treatment, vector control and social mobilization. In 2005, a memorandum of understanding was signed by Bangladesh, India and Nepal to overcome anthroponotic visceral Leishmaniasis by reducing the incidence of the disease to <1 case/10 000 population by 2015 (*12*).

Endemic countries in East Africa will follow revised national guidelines and rely mainly on combination treatment for visceral Leishmaniasis (sodium stibogluconate and paromomycin). Combination therapy has reduced the duration and cost of treatment, improved patients' adherence, and is expected to delay or even prevent drug resistance. To control cutaneous Leishmaniasis, WHO's Eastern Mediterranean Region, which has the highest burden of the disease, has developed a 5-year strategic plan and case-management guidelines in consultation with other countries where the disease is endemic.

Controlling vectors and reservoir hosts is important for controlling the Leishmaniases. Countries should regularly monitor and assess the effectiveness of different strategies being used for vector control, including indoor residual spraying with insecticides and the use of treated bednets.

REFERENCES

[1]   *Control of the Leishmaniases*. Geneva, World Health Organization, 2010 (WHO Technical Report Series, No. 949).

[2]   Alvar J et al. Leishmaniasis worldwide and global estimates of its incidence. *PLoS One*, 2012, 7(5): e35671 (doi:10.1371/journal.pone.0035671).

[3]   Desjeux P. Worldwide increasing risk factors for leishmaniasis. *Medical Microbiology and Immunology*, 2001, 190:77–79.

[4]   Aagaard-Hansen J et al. Population movement: a key factor in the epidemiology of neglected tropical diseases. *Tropical Medicine and International Health*, 2010, 15:1281–1288.

[5]   Alvar J et al. The relationship between leishmaniasis and AIDS: the second 10 years. *Clinical Microbiology Reviews*, 2008, 21:334–359.

[6]   Reithinger R et al. Anthroponotic cutaneous leishmaniasis, Kabul, Afghanistan. *Emerging Infectious Diseases*, 2003, 9:727–729.

[7]   *Upsurge of kala-azar in South Sudan requires rapid response*. Geneva, World Health Organization, 2010 (http://www.who.int/leishmaniasis/Upsurge_kalaazar_Southern_Sudan.pdf; accessed November 2012).

[8]   Sharma DA et al. The economic impact of visceral leishmaniasis on households in Bangladesh. *Tropical Medicine and International Health*, 2006, 11:757–764.

[9]   Sarnoff R et al. The economic impact of visceral leishmaniasis in rural households in one endemic district of Bihar, India. *Tropical Medicine and International Health*, 2010, 15(Suppl. 2): S42–49.

[10] *Resolution WHA60.13: control of leishmaniasis*. Geneva, World Health Assembly, 2007.

[11] *Report of a WHO informal consultation on liposomal amphotericin B in the treatment of visceral leishmaniasis*. Geneva, World Health Organization, 2005 (WHO/CDS/NTD/IDM/2007.4).

[12] *Regional strategic framework for elimination of kala-azar from the South-East Asia Region (2005–2015)*. New Delhi, World Health Organization, Regional Office for South-East Asia (SEA-VBC-85, Rev. 1).

DISEASES

3.10   TAENIASIS/CYSTICERCOSIS

Introduction

Taeniasis and cysticercosis are caused by infection with the tapeworm *Taenia solium*. The presence of the adult tapeworm in the intestine causes taeniasis, a mildly pathogenic disease. Conversely, cysticercosis is a severe disease that results when humans ingest the tapeworm's eggs, and larvae (cysticerci) develop in their tissues. Cysticerci may develop in muscles, skin, the eyes and the central nervous system. Neurocysticercosis is the term used when the central nervous system is invaded.

Taeniasis and cysticercosis are closely interrelated: cysticercosis can infect pigs, and consumption of infected pork is responsible for taeniasis in humans.

The intermittent release of tapeworm eggs in the faeces of humans with taeniasis contaminates the environment and exposes humans and pigs to the risk of infection with cystercercosis.

Distribution

The distribution of disease caused by infection with *T. solium* has changed little since 2010. Endemic regions include Latin America, South Asia and South-East Asia, and

Fig. 3.10.1 Global distribution of cysticercosis, 2011

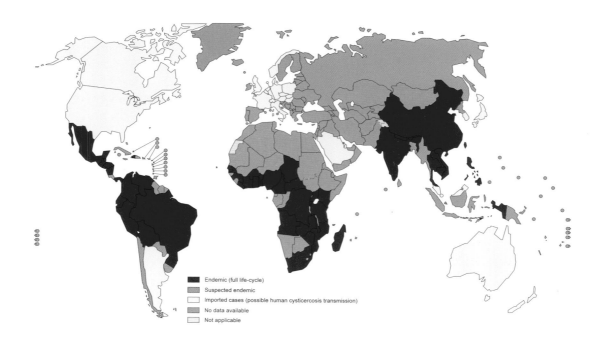

Endemic (full life-cycle)
Suspected endemic
Imported cases (possible human cysticercosis transmission)
No data available
Not applicable

sub-Saharan Africa (*Fig. 3.10.1*). High prevalences of human cysticercosis occur in various foci in Burkina Faso, the Democratic Republic of the Congo, Mozambique, Senegal, South Africa, the United Republic of Tanzania and Zambia. In Asia, new reports of cases of neurocysticercosis have been received from Bangladesh, Malaysia and Singapore, mainly in migrant workers.

Impact

Neurocysticercosis is responsible for the largest burden caused by *T. solium*-associated diseases, and is probably the most frequent preventable cause of epilepsy in developing countries (*Table 3.10.1*). Among people with epilepsy in endemic countries, the proportion who had neurocysticercosis has been estimated to be 29% (*1*). WHO estimates that at least 50 million people worldwide have epilepsy, and that about one third of all cases occur in regions where *T. solium* infection is endemic (*2*).

Table 3.10.1 Estimated number of cases of cysticercosis and cases of epilepsy associated with neurocysticercosis, by geographical area (*3,4*)

Area	No. of human cysticercosis cases	No. of active epilepsy cases associated with neurocysticercosis
Africa	ND	0.31 million to 4.6 million
China	3 million to 6 million	ND
India	ND	> 1 million
Latin America	11 million to 29 million	0.45 million to 1.35 million
Mexico	ND	144 433

ND, no data available

Neurocysticercosis may be fatal, and it has been reported as a cause of death in Brazil (*5*), Cameroon (*6*), Mexico (*5*) and the United States of America (*7*). The annual proportion of deaths caused by epilepsy associated with neurocysticercosis has been estimated to be 6.9% of incident cases in Cameroon and 0.5% in Mexico (*5,6*).

In Peru, the costs of treatment and losses in productivity caused by neurocysticercosis consume 54% of the total annual minimum wage during the first year of treatment, and account for 16% during the second year. Symptoms of neurocysticercosis cause an average loss of 44.5 hours of productive activity per month. The symptoms of cysticercosis cause two thirds of wage-earners to lose their jobs, and only 61% are able to again engage in wage-earning activities (*8*).

Porcine cysticercosis has a serious impact on pig-producing communities. It leads to poor quality pork, which causes prices to fall or pork to be condemned as unfit for consumption, thereby reducing income and making an important source of protein unsafe to consume.

In a field trial in Cameroon, the porcine cysticercosis vaccine (*9*) and a single treatment of pigs with oxfendazole eliminated transmission of *T. solium* (*10*). The vaccine prevents new larval infection in pigs but does not affect established cysticerci, hence the need to treat with oxfendazole to eliminate them from muscles, which produces a positive impact on human health. A commercial process for producing the vaccine has been developed, and registration trials are continuing. Simultaneous safety and bioequivalence studies are in progress to provide formulations of oxfendazole that will be registered for use in pigs.

Strategy (roadmap targets and milestones)

Cysticercosis, neurocysticercosis and taeniasis were added by WHO to the list of neglected tropical diseases in 2010. An interagency meeting held in 2011 by WHO, FAO, OIE and other experts to plan for preventing and controlling neglected zoonotic diseases highlighted cysticercosis, neurocysticercosis and taeniasis as diseases of global importance. Participants at the meeting estimated that US$ 2 million would be needed annually to support initial pilot projects for implementing national programmes (*11*). Medium-term and long-term needs include validating a strategy for controlling and eliminating *T. solium* cysticercosis, neurocysticercosis and taeniasis by 2015, and then using the validated strategy to scale up interventions in selected endemic countries by 2020 (*12*). WHO and its partners are committed to attaining these milestones by improving tools for control, and formulating best-practice guidelines for interrupting transmission; the guidelines and tools will be pilot tested in selected endemic areas.

An appropriate, standard methodology for intervention needs to be developed and validated in endemic communities. Information suggests that it is insufficient to implement a single approach to controlling diseases caused by *T. solium* (*13*). Intervention studies in Honduras and Peru have shown that transmission can be interrupted and that an important cause of epilepsy can be reduced in resource-constrained, endemic countries (*14,15*). Elimination will require (i) improvements in chemotherapy for humans and pigs, (ii) routine vaccination of pigs in endemic areas, (iii) better management of pig farms and pork production practices, (iv) improved sanitation, and (v) health education.

DISEASES

REFERENCES

[1]   Ndimubanzi PC et al. A systematic review of the frequency of neurocyticercosis with a focus on people with epilepsy. *PLoS Neglected Tropical Diseases*, 2010, 4(11): e870 (doi:10.1371/journal.pntd.0000870).

[2]   *Atlas: epilepsy care in the world 2005*. Geneva, World Health Organization, 2005.

[3]   Bhattarai R et al. Estimating the non-monetary burden of neurocysticercosis in Mexico. *PLoS Neglected Tropical Diseases*, 2012, 6:e1521 (doi:10.1371/journal.pntd.0001521).

[4]   Coyle CM et al. Neurocysticercosis: neglected but not forgotten. *PLoS Neglected Tropical Diseases*, 2012, 6:e1500.

[5]   Santo AH. Tendência da mortalidade relacionada à cisticercose no Estado de São Paulo, Brasil, 1985 a 2004: estudo usando causas múltiplas de morte [Cysticercosis-related mortality in the State of São Paulo, Brazil, 1985–2004: a study using multiple causes of death]. *Cadernos de Saúde Pública*, 2007, 23:2917–2927.

[6]   Praet N et al. The disease burden of *Taenia solium* cysticercosis in Cameroon. *PLoS Neglected Tropical Diseases*, 2009, 3:e406 (doi:10.1371/journal.pntd.0000406).

[7]   Holmes NE et al. Neurocysticercosis causing sudden death. *American Journal of Forensic Medicine and Pathology*, 2010, 31:117–119.

[8]   Rajkotia Y et al. Economic burden of cysticercosis: results from Peru. *Transactions of the Royal Society of Tropical Medicine and Hygiene*, 2007, 101:840–846.

[9]   Lightowlers MW. Eradication of *Taenia solium* cysticercosis: a role for vaccination of pigs. *International Journal for Parasitology*, 2010, 40:1183–1192.

[10] Assana E et al. Elimination of *Taenia solium* transmission to pigs in a field trial of the TSOL18 vaccine in Cameroon. *International Journal for Parasitology*, 2010, 40:515–519.

[11] *The interagency meeting on planning the prevention and control of neglected zoonotic diseases (NZDs)*. Geneva, World Health Organization, 2011 (WHO/HTM/NTD/NZD/2011.3).

[12] *Accelerating work to overcome the global impact of neglected tropical diseases: a roadmap for implementation*. Geneva, World Health Organization, 2012 (WHO/HTM/NTD/2012.1).

[13] *Report of the WHO expert consultation on foodborne trematode infections and taeniasis/cysticercosis*. Geneva, World Health Organization, 2011 (WHO/HTM/NTD/PCT/2011.3).

[14] Garcia HH et al. Epidemiología y control de la cisticercosis en el Perú [Epidemiology and control of cysticercosis in Peru]. *Revista Peruana de Medicina Experimental y Salud Pública*, 2010, 27:592–597.

[15] Medina MT et al. Reduction in rate of epilepsy from neurocysticercosis by community interventions: the Salamá, Honduras study. *Epilepsia*, 2011, 52:1177–1185.

3.11 DRACUNCULIASIS (GUINEA-WORM DISEASE)

Introduction

Dracunculiasis is approaching eradication (*1*). The disease results from infection with the nematode *Dracunculus medinensis*, the guinea worm. People become infected by drinking water containing infected cyclopoid copepods (Crustacea). No medicine or vaccine is effective in curing or preventing the disease: eradication is being achieved by implementing public-health measures.

Distribution

During the 1980s, dracunculiasis was endemic in 20 countries in WHO's African, Eastern Mediterranean and South-East Asia regions. In 1989, a total of 892 055 cases in 13 682 villages were reported from the 15 countries that submitted reports from the village level (*2*). This change is shown in *Fig. 3.11.1*. By the end of 2012, dracunculiasis was limited to four countries where the disease is endemic and a total of 542 cases in 271 villages; 521 (96%) of these cases were reported in 254 villages in South Sudan, 10 cases were reported in Chad, and 4 each in Ethiopia and Mali

Fig. 3.11.1 Countries endemic for dracunculiasis, 1989 and 2012

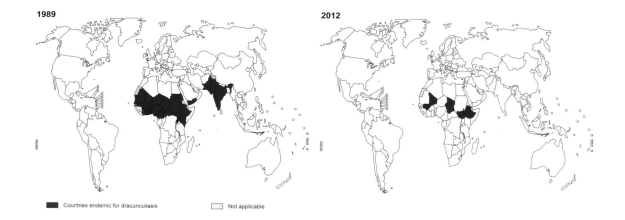

(provisional data). Niger, currently in the precertification stage, reported 3 imported cases from Mali. The steady decline in the monthly number of cases is shown in *Fig. 3.11.2*.

Fig. 3.11.2 Number of dracunculiasis cases reported to WHO, by month, 2010–2012

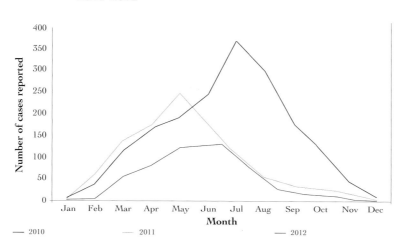

ᵃ Data for 2012 are provisional up to December.

Impact

Eradicating dracunculiasis ensures that people will be spared burning pain as worms emerge from their body; worms most commonly emerge from the lower limbs. People will also be spared reduced mobility from inflamed ankles and knees caused by worms emerging near these joints. The worst effects on mobility invariably coincide with harvest time. In 1987, a study in Nigeria estimated an annual loss of US$ 20 million per single crop (rice, yam or cassava) from farmers incapacitated by the disease for an average duration of 5 weeks (*3–5*).

The eradication of dracunculiasis is estimated to lead to a 29% increase in economic return for the agricultural sector of countries where the disease is no longer endemic (*6*).

Strategy (roadmap targets and milestones)

The eradication strategy recommended by WHO and adopted by all national programmes combines the following approaches: (i) improving surveillance; (ii) intensifying case-containment measures; (iii) providing access to improved drinking-water sources; (iv) controlling vectors by treating potential sources of unsafe water with temephos (Abate) and distributing filters to strain water; and (v) promoting behavioural change and awareness by providing information and education. Once a country claims to have interrupted transmission, by reporting zero indigenous cases for at least 3 years, it becomes eligible for certification of eradication through a process recommended by the International Commission for the Certification of Dracunculiasis Eradication (7).

Progress towards global eradication has been impressive. By May 2010, Ghana had interrupted transmission and is now in the precertification stage. Transmission was not interrupted in Ethiopia and Mali by 2011 although this had been anticipated. Chad, a country in the precertification stage, experienced an outbreak in 2010, more than 10 years after reporting its last known case in 2000. In Chad, 10 cases were reported in 2010, another 10 cases in 2011 and 10 new cases in 2012 reverting to endemic country status. Investigation revealed that surveillance may have failed to detect recent cases (1,8). After South Sudan became independent in July 2011, Sudan entered the precertification stage because its last indigenous case was reported in 2002.

In 2011, the World Health Assembly in resolution 64.16 called on Member States already certified as free of dracunculiasis or those in the precertification stage to intensify surveillance (1). Surveillance was carried out through house to house surveys during national immunization days in the 10 countries where the disease is endemic or that are in the precertification stage, with the exception of South Sudan. In 2011, WHO's Regional Office for Africa issued instructions to its country offices to assist in integrating surveillance for dracunculiasis with that for polio (1).

A monetary reward for voluntarily reporting of cases is in place in all endemic countries, including those in the precertification stage, except South Sudan. The scheme is working. By 2011, the reward was associated with the reporting of 21/30 cases outside of South Sudan, with 10/10 cases in Chad, with 6/ 8 in Ethiopia, and with 5/12 in Mali. In 2010, rewards were paid for the reporting of 73/ 88 cases outside of southern Sudan, 10/10 in Chad, 18/21 in Ethiopia, and 45/57 in Mali.

Between 1995 and 2012, the International Commission for the Certification of Dracunculiasis Eradication met eight times and, on the basis of its recommendations, WHO has been able to certify 192 countries, territories and areas of 180 Member States as being free from dracunculiasis, either by having interrupted transmission or by being an area where transmission is never known to have occurred. The status of all countries by endemicity and certification stage is shown in *Fig.3.11.3*.

Fig. 3.11.3 Status of global certification of dracunculiasis eradication, 2012

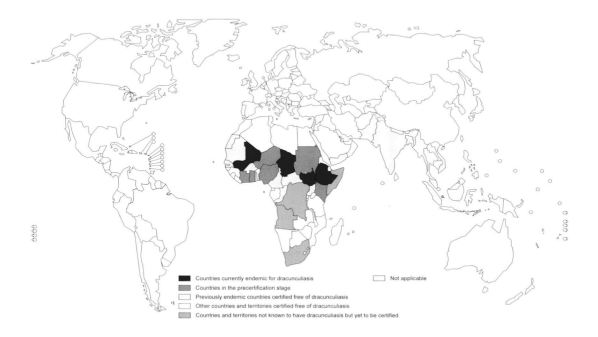

Countries currently endemic for dracunculiasis

Countries in the precertification stage

Previously endemic countries certified free of dracunculiasis

Other countries and territories certified free of dracunculiasis

Countries and territories not known to have dracunculiasis but yet to be certified

Not applicable

The roadmap's target for eradication (*Table 3.11.1*) should be achieved provided that various challenges are overcome. The reasons why cases occurred in Chad and certain areas of Mali are not yet understood. Surveillance systems need to be improved, and improvements sustained, to meet the standard of exhaustively detecting indigenous transmission and imported cases. In South Sudan, the identification of transmission sources in remaining foci remains problematic owing to population movement and insecurity. Recurring insecurity in Mali is of concern to that country's national eradication effort. Of the five regions in Mali where dracunculiasis was endemic in 2012, the eradication programme was not fully operating in two provinces (Gao and Timbuktu); additionally, the programme was unable to carry out interventions in the region of Kidal. Surveillance has been intensified in the Malian refugee camps in Burkina Faso, Mauritania and Niger in an effort to prevent the spread of infection and disease. Similarly, the Ethiopian dracunculiasis eradication programme is reinforcing surveillance in areas bordering South Sudan.

DISEASES

Table 3.11.1 Milestones for eradicating dracunculiasis

Milestones	2013	2014	2015
Countries where transmission has been interrupted	Ethiopia	Chad, Mali	South Sudan
No. of countries certified	183 Member States	183 Member States	190 Member States

According to WHO and The Carter Center, the final drive towards eradication will need US$ 62 million during 2011–2015. The Government of the United Kingdom has pledged up to £20 million; the Bill & Melinda Gates Foundation has confirmed it will provide an additional US$ 23.3 million; the remaining amount will be provided by the government of the United Arab Emirates (US$ 10 million) and the Children's Investment Fund Foundation (US$ 6.7 million).

REFERENCES

[1]　Dracunculiasis eradication – global surveillance summary, 2011. *Weekly Epidemiological Record*, 2012, 87: 177–188.

[2]　Dracunculiasis – global surveillance summary, 1992. *Weekly Epidemiological Record*, 1993, 68:125–131.

[3]　Dracunculiasis: global surveillance summary, 1987. *Weekly Epidemiological Record*, 1988, 49:375–378.

[4]　Hopkins DR et al. Dracunculiasis eradication: delayed, not denied. *American Journal of Tropical Medicine and Hygiene*, 2000, 62:163–168.

[5]　Rooy C de. *Guinea worm control as a major contributor to self-sufficiency in rice production in Nigeria*. Lagos, Nigeria, UNICEF Water, Environment and Sanitation Section, 1987.

[6]　Jim A, Tandon A, Ruiz-Tiben E. *Cost-benefit analysis of the global dracunculiasis eradication campaign*. Washington DC, World Bank, 1997 (Policy Research Working Paper No. 1835).

[7]　*Certification of dracunculiasis eradication: criteria, strategies, procedures*. Geneva, World Health Organization, 1996.

[8]　Renewed transmission of dracunculiasis – Chad, 2010. *Morbidity and Mortality Weekly Report*, 2011, 60; 744–748.

3.12   ECHINOCOCCOSIS

Introduction

Echinococcosis is recognized as one of the neglected zoonotic diseases (*1*). Human echinococcosis is a parasitic disease that occurs in two main forms: cystic echinococcosis (hydatidosis), caused by infection with *Echinococcus granulosus*, and alveolar echinococcosis, caused by infection with *E. multilocularis*. Both organisms are tapeworms and their definitive hosts, which harbour the adult parasite in their intestines, are domestic and wild carnivores. The intermediate hosts, which harbour the larval stages of the parasite, are a number of farm animals and wild ungulates, rodents, and other small mammals. Humans are accidental intermediate hosts. *Echinococcus* eggs are most commonly shed in faeces of dogs and several wild canids, such as foxes, wolves, jackals and coyotes.

When humans become infected by ingesting *Echinococcus* eggs, the lesions characteristic of each form begin to develop. Human infection with *E. granulosus* leads to the development of one or several fluid-filled cysts (hydatid cysts) that are surrounded by a capsule of host origin; these are located mainly in the liver and lungs, and less frequently in other body districts including the bones, kidneys, spleen, muscles, central nervous system and behind the eye. The incubation period can last many years, with signs and symptoms depending on the location of the cyst, or cysts, and the pressure exerted on the surrounding tissues and organs. Infection with *E. multilocularis* leads to the formation of a multivesiculated tumour, mainly in the liver (*2,3*). Alveolar echinococcosis is characterized by an asymptomatic incubation period of 5–15 years. Larval metastases may form in organs adjacent to the liver or in distant locations following dissemination of the parasite by the haematogenous or lymphatic route.

Distribution

The global distribution of cystic echinococcosis has changed little since 2010 (*Fig. 3.12.1*). Highly endemic areas are mostly found in the eastern part of the Mediterranean region, northern Africa, southern and eastern Europe, at the southern tip of South America, in Central Asia, Siberia and western China. Alveolar echinococcosis is confined to the northern hemisphere, in particular to regions of China, The Russian Federation and countries in continental Europe and North America. Both diseases are considered to be underreported; however, data indicate that echinococcosis is re-emerging as an important public health problem. There are more than 1 million people worldwide affected with these diseases at any one time (*4,5*).

Fig. 3.12.1 Global distribution of cystic echinococcosis, 2011

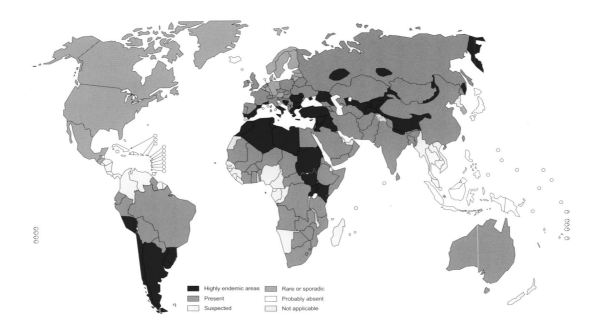

Highly endemic areas   Rare or sporadic
Present   Probably absent
Suspected   Not applicable

Impact

The annual costs associated with cystic echinococcosis are estimated to be US$ 3 billion, which includes costs for treating cases and losses to the livestock industry (*4*). In humans, echinococcosis can be life-threatening if undiagnosed and untreated. Treatment for cystic echinococcosis and alveolar echinococcosis often includes surgery. In regions where cystic echinococcosis is endemic, the incidence in humans can exceed 50/100 000 person-years; prevalences as high as 5–10% may occur in parts of Argentina, Central Asia, China, East Africa and Peru (*6*). The postoperative death rate for surgical patients is 2.2%; 6.5% of cases relapse after intervention and require prolonged recovery time (*4*). In certain communities on the Tibetan Plateau of China, there may be as many as 5-10% of the population infected with *E. multilocularis*, and the annual incidence of cases of alveolar echinococcosis possibly exceeds 16 000 in this region (*5*).

In livestock, the rate of cystic echinococcosis found in slaughterhouses in hyperendemic areas of Latin America varies from 20% to 95% of slaughtered animals. The highest rates have been found in rural areas where older animals are slaughtered (*7*). In Sardinia, Italy, during 2005–2010 in the absence of specific control measures, the prevalence of cystic echinococcosis in sheep was 65%, with about 14% of sheep harbouring at least one fertile cyst (*8*). Livestock production losses attributable to cystic echinococcosis depend on which species is infected but include the liver being condemned as unfit for consumption, a reduction in the weight of carcasses, a decrease in the value of the animal's hide, a decrease in milk production and reduced fecundity (*4*).

Strategy (roadmap targets and milestones)

By 2015, pilot projects for validating effective strategies for controlling cystic echinococcosis will be under way in selected countries. Validated strategies for controlling the disease, and integrated control packages for major dog-related zoonoses (rabies and echinococcosis), will be available in 2018. Large-scale interventions for controlling and eliminating cystic echinococcosis as a public-health problem in selected countries will be initiated on that basis and will be continued through 2020. The cost of implementing these pilot projects in three countries during 2013–2017 has been estimated to be about US$ 10 million over 5 years (*9*).

WHO's informal working group on echinococcosis has developed consensus about treating human cystic echinococcosis and alveolar echinococcosis (*5*). Four options exist for cystic echinococcosis: (i) percutaneous treatments including puncture, aspiration, injection, and re-aspiration (known as PAIR); (ii) surgery; (iii) treatment with anti-infective medicines; or (iv) watch and wait. The choice must primarily be made based on the results of ultrasound imaging of the cyst that follows a stage-specific approach. It also depends on the medical infrastructure and human resources available. An agreement has recently been signed between WHO and the Italian Ministry of Health to decentralize diagnostic and therapeutic techniques and promote the PAIR strategy, where indicated, for managing cystic echinococcosis in rural, hyperendemic areas of Morocco and Tunisia.

For alveolar echinococcosis, the key elements for treatment of human cases remain early diagnosis and radical (tumour-like) surgery followed by anti-infective prophylaxis with albendazole. If the lesion is confined, radical surgery offers cure.

Cystic echinococcosis is preventable because it involves domesticated animal species as definitive and intermediate hosts. Periodically treating dogs, ensuring control measures in the slaughter of livestock with safe destruction of contaminated offal, and engaging in public education have been found to lower transmission, and to prevent it in wealthy countries. In endemic areas, the health sector often takes the lead in initiating echinococcosis-control measures, but it is dependent on the veterinary sector for animal-related interventions. Vaccinating sheep with an *E. granulosus* recombinant oncosphere antigen (EG95) offers encouraging prospects for prevention and control. Small-scale EG95 vaccine trials in sheep indicate that it has high efficacy and safety in vaccinated lambs, and they do not become infected with

E. granulosus (*10*). A programme combining the vaccination of lambs, treatment of dogs, and culling of older sheep could lead to disease elimination in humans in less than 10 years (*8*).

Preventing and controlling alveolar echinococcosis are more complex because the organism's life-cycle involves wild animal species as definitive and intermediate hosts. Regular deworming of domestic carnivores that have access to wild rodents should help reduce the risk of infection to humans. Deworming of wild and stray definitive hosts with anthelminthic baits resulted in drastic reductions in prevalence in Europe (*2,11*) and Japan (*12*).

REFERENCES

[1] *The control of neglected zoonotic diseases: community-based interventions for prevention and control.* Geneva, World Health Organization, 2011 (WHO/HTM/NTD/NZD/2011.1).

[2] *Report of a WHO informal working group on cystic and alveolar echinococcosis surveillance, prevention and control, with the participation of the Food and Agriculture Organization of the United Nations and the World Organisation for Animal Health.* Geneva, World Health Organization, 2011 (WHO/HTM/NTD/NZD/2011.2).

[3] Brunetti E et al. Expert consensus for the diagnosis and treatment of cystic and alveolar echinococcosis in humans. *Acta Tropica*, 2010, 114:1–16.

[4] Budke C et al. Global socioeconomic impact of cystic echinococcosis. *Emerging Infectious Diseases*, 2006, 12:296–302.

[5] Torgerson PR et al. The global burden of alveolar echinococcosis. *PLoS Neglected Tropical Diseases*, 2010, 4:e722 (doi:10.1371/journal.pntd.0000722).

[6] Craig P et al. Prevention and control of cystic echinococcosis. *Lancet Infectious Diseases*, 2007, 7:385–394.

[7] *Zoonoses and communicable diseases common to man and animals*, vol. III, 3rd ed. Washington, DC, Pan American Health Organization, 2001 (Scientific and Technical Publication No. 580).

[8] Conchedda M et al. Cystic echinococcosis in sheep in Sardinia. Changing pattern and present status. *Acta Tropica*, 2012, 122:52–58.

[9] *The interagency meeting on planning the prevention and control of neglected zoonotic diseases (NZDs).* Geneva, World Health Organization, 2011 (WHO/HTM/NTD/NZD/2011.3).

[10] Lightowlers M et al. Vaccination against cysticercosis and hydatid disease. *Parasitology Today*, 2000, 16:191–196.

[11] Hegglin D, Deplazes P. Control strategy for *Echinococcus multilocularis*. *Emerging Infectious Diseases*, 2008, 14:1626–1628.

[12] Tsukada H et al. Potential remedy against *Echinococcus multilocularis* in wild red foxes using baits with anthelminthic distributed around fox breeding dens in Hokkaido, Japan. *Parasitology*, 2002, 125:119–129.

3.13 FOODBORNE TREMATODIASES

Introduction

Infections with foodborne trematodes are acquired when food contaminated with larval stages of metacercariae is ingested. The diseases of most public-health importance are clonorchiasis (caused by infection with *Clonorchis sinensis*), opisthorchiasis (infection with *Opisthorchis viverrini* or *O. felineus*), fascioliasis (infection with *Fasciola hepatica* or *F. gigantica*), and paragonimiasis (infection with *Paragonimus* spp.) (*Table 3.13.1*).

Table 3.13.1 Epidemiological characteristics of most common foodborne trematodiases

Disease	Infectious agent	Acquired through consumption of	Natural final host	Primary organ affected
Clonorchiasis	*Clonorchis sinensis*	Fish	Dogs and other fish-eating carnivores	Liver
Opisthorchiasis	*Opisthorchis viverrini; O. felineus*	Fish	Cats and other fish-eating carnivores	Liver
Fascioliasis	*Fasciola hepatica; F. gigantica*	Vegetables	Sheep, cattle and other herbivores	Liver
Paragonimiasis	*Paragonimus* spp.	Crustaceans (crabs and crayfish)	Cats, dogs and other crustacean-eating carnivores	Lungs

Distribution

Although cases of foodborne trematodiases have been reported from more than 70 countries worldwide, countries in Asia and Latin America are the most badly affected (*1*). Information on the epidemiological status of foodborne trematodes in Africa is limited, but paragonimiasis is known to be transmitted in the central and western parts of the continent. Estimates limited to 17 countries indicate that in 2005 there were more than 56 million infected individuals, 7.9 million had severe sequelae, and more than 7000 had died from infection with foodborne trematodes (*1*) (*Figs. 3.13.1– 3.13.4*).

Morbidity due to infection with foodborne trematodes is both systemic and organ-specific, and becomes more severe as the number of worms increases through subsequent rounds of infection. Chronic infections with *C. sinensis* and *O. viverrini* are strongly associated with cholangiocarcinoma. Both parasites are classified by the International Agency for Research on Cancer as carcinogenic to humans (*2*).

The economic burden of foodborne trematodes is mainly linked to the expanding livestock and aquaculture industries. Losses in animal production and trade are likely to indirectly affect human welfare. Although estimates are not available, their projected impact is nevertheless significant.

Fig. 3.13.1 Global distribution of clonorchiasis, latest year available (modified from (*3*))

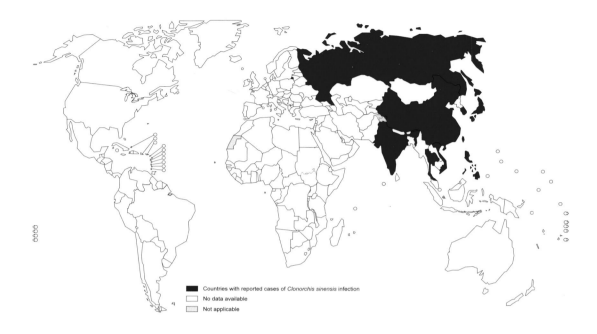

Countries with reported cases of *Clonorchis sinensis* infection
No data available
Not applicable

Fig. 3.13.2 Global distribution of opisthorchiasis, latest year available (modified from (*3*))

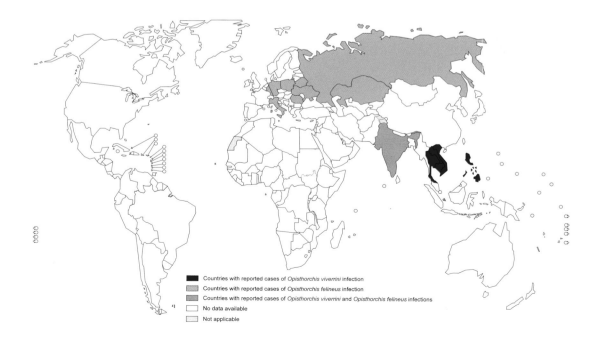

Countries with reported cases of *Opisthorchis viverrini* infection
Countries with reported cases of *Opisthorchis felineus* infection
Countries with reported cases of *Opisthorchis viverrini* and *Opisthorchis felineus* infections
No data available
Not applicable

Fig. 3.13.3 Global distribution of fascioliasis, latest year available (modified from (3))

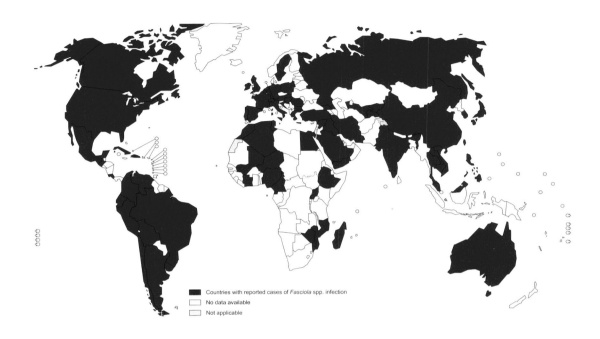

■ Countries with reported cases of *Fasciola* spp. infection
□ No data available
□ Not applicable

Fig. 3.13.4 Global distribution of paragonimiasis, latest year available (modified from (3))

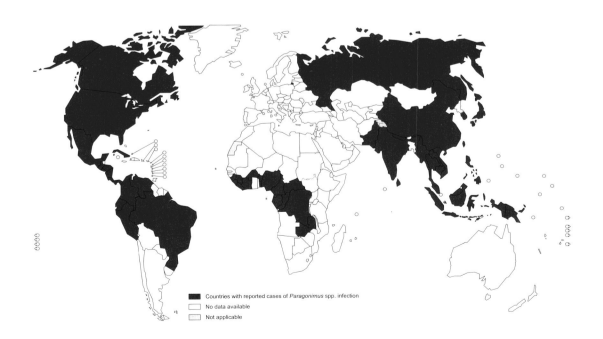

■ Countries with reported cases of *Paragonimus* spp. infection
□ No data available
□ Not applicable

Strategy (roadmap targets and milestones)

A public-health strategy to combat foodborne trematodiases has been developed in the past few years (3). Its mainstay is treatment of the human host, with the aim of controlling morbidity and ultimately preventing associated mortality. The objective is to ensure that medicines are available to treat those who need them. Praziquantel is the treatment of choice for clonorchiasis and opisthorchiasis, and triclabendazole for fascioliasis; either medicine can also be used to treat paragonimiasis. Treatment strategies vary, from individual case-management to the mass delivery of preventive chemotherapy.

Praziquantel has been used as preventive chemotherapy for approximately 30 years. By contrast, delivering triclabendazole as preventive chemotherapy to all individuals in a community had not been undertaken until 2008, when the ministries of health of the Plurinational State of Bolivia and Peru decided to conduct pilot studies in areas where people were at high risk of fascioliasis. Results from both countries confirmed the efficacy and safety of this approach (*Table 3.13.2*) (*4,5*).

Table 3.13.2 Recommended treatments and strategies to control foodborne trematodiases

Disease	Recommended medicine and dose	Recommended strategy	
Clonorchiasis and Opisthorchiasis	Praziquantel • 40 mg/kg single administration, or • 25 mg/kg 3 times daily for 2–3 consecutive days	Preventive chemotherapy • Treat all residents in districts where prevalence of infection is ≥20% once every 12 months • Treat all residents in districts where prevalence of infection is < 20% once every 24 months or treat only the individuals who report regularly eating raw fish every 12 months	
Fascioliasis	Triclabendazole • 10 mg/kg single administration	Individual case-management • Treat all confirmed cases • In endemic areas treat all suspected cases Preventive chemotherapy • In subdistricts, villages or communities where cases of fascioliasis are clustered treat all school-aged children (5–14 years) or all residents once every 12 months	
Paragonimiasis	Triclabendazole • 2 doses of 10 mg/kg delivered on the same day (individual case-management) or • 20 mg/kg single administration (preventive chemotherapy) Praziquantel • 25 mg/kg 3 times daily for 3 days (individual case-management)	Individual case-management • Treat all confirmed cases • In endemic areas treat all suspected cases Preventive chemotherapy • In subdistricts, villages or communities where cases of paragonimiasis are clustered treat all residents once every 12 months	

Although millions of people in Thailand have been screened and treated, opisthorchiasis is still the most prevalent helminth infection there. In 2012, the number of affected individuals exceeded 6 million; most of those affected live in the north-eastern provinces (6). More than 5000 new cases of cholangiocarcinoma, most of which are fatal, are diagnosed annually in Thailand (7).

In the Lao People's Democratic Republic, about 2 million people are estimated to have opisthorchiasis (6). Preventive chemotherapy with praziquantel started in 2007, and in 2011 approximately 325 000 children and adults were treated.

In Viet Nam, preventive chemotherapy with praziquantel started in 2006, and in 2011 more than 128 000 people were treated for clonorchiasis. In the Republic of Korea, in 2011 approximately 4000 people were treated for clonorchiasis in the remaining endemic areas.

In Cambodia, mapping continues in an effort to identify areas where foodborne trematodes are transmitted. It is estimated that at least 600 000 people are infected with *O. viverrini* (5,6), and implementation of pilot control interventions based on WHO's recommendations is planned.

In South America, the Plurinational State of Bolivia is engaged in the largest fascioliasis-control programme worldwide. The population requiring preventive chemotherapy is estimated to be 250 000 children and adults. Since 2008, more than 540 000 doses of triclabendazole have been administered. Peru is also engaged in scaling up its control programme by providing preventive chemotherapy in high-priority districts.

In Egypt, programmes to control fascioliasis started in 1998 in the Nile Delta, where the infected population has been estimated to be 830 000. Since 1998, widespread control activities have been carried out in endemic villages where intestinal schistosomiasis also occurs. The prevalence of human fascioliasis has steadily decreased. In 2011, several hundred infected children and adults were identified and treated with triclabendazole.

Two implementation milestones have been set for foodborne trematodiases. By 2015, WHO aims to support endemic countries to help them control morbidity associated with these diseases. By 2020, the aim is to ensure that at least 75% of the worldwide population requiring preventive chemotherapy has been reached (8).

Ensuring that medicines are available is the key to reaching the roadmap's targets. Triclabendazole has been donated to treat fascioliasis and paragonimiasis, but access to praziquantel to treat clonorchiasis and opisthorchiasis has not been secured. A rough estimate of the need in Cambodia, the Lao People's Democratic Republic and Viet Nam ranges from 10 million to 15 million 600 mg tablets of praziquantel per year.

REFERENCES

[1] Fürst T et al. Global burden of human food-borne trematodiasis: a systematic review and meta-analysis. *Lancet Infectious Diseases*, 2012, 12:210–221.

[2] *A review of human carcinogens. Biological agents. IARC Monographs on the evaluation of carcinogenic risks to humans*. Volume 100 B. Lyon, World Health Organization, 2012.

[3] *Report of the WHO expert consultation on foodborne trematode infections and taeniasis/cysticercosis.* Geneva, World Health Organization, 2011 (WHO/HTM/NTD/PCT/2011.3).

[4] Villegas F et al. Administration of triclabendazole is safe and effective in controlling fascioliasis in an endemic community of the Bolivian Altiplano. *PLoS Neglected Tropical Diseases*, 2012, 6:e1720 (doi:10.1371/journal.pntd.0001720).

[5] Ortiz P. Estado actual de la infección por *Fasciola hepática* en Cajamarca, Perú [Current status of *Fasciola hepatica* infection in Cajamarca, Peru]. *Biomédica*, 2011, 31(Suppl. 3):S172–S173.

[6] Sithithaworn P et al. The current status of opisthorchiasis and clonorchiasis in the Mekong basin. *Parasitology International*, 2012, 61:10–16.

[7] Scripa B et al. Opisthorchiasis and *Opisthorchis*-associated cholangiocarcinoma in Thailand and Laos. *Acta Tropica*, 2011, 120(Suppl 1):S158–168.

[8] *Accelerating work to overcome the global impact of neglected tropical diseases: a roadmap for implementation.* Geneva, World Health Organization, 2012 (WHO/HTM/NTD/2012.1).

3.14   LYMPHATIC FILARIASIS

Introduction

Lymphatic filariasis is caused by infection with one of three species of filarial nematode, *Wuchereria bancrofti*, *Brugia malayi* or *B. timori*, which are transmitted by mosquitoes. Adult worms live almost exclusively in humans, and lodge in the lymphatic system. The infection is commonly acquired during childhood but usually manifests during adulthood.

Distribution

Mapping the distribution of lymphatic filariasis has progressed rapidly during the past decade, so reliable data are available about how many people need treatment and how many have received treatment. Globally, 1.39 billion people require preventive chemotherapy, and 70/72 endemic countries have initiated programmes to eliminate lymphatic filariasis. WHO's South-East Asia and African regions have the highest numbers of people requiring preventive treatment: 877 million people in 9 countries (63%) in the South-East Asia Region require preventive treatment, as do 432 million people in 34 countries (31%) in the Africa Region. The Mekong Plus area (6 endemic countries: Brunei Darussalam, Cambodia, the Lao People's Democratic Republic, Malaysia, the Philippines and Viet Nam) accounts for 3% of the global population needing preventive treatment; the Region of the Americas (4 endemic countries), the Eastern Mediterranean Region (3 endemic countries) and Oceania (16 endemic countries) account for another 3% (*1*).

Brugia infections are confined to WHO's South-East Asia Region.

In 2011, the Strategic and Technical Advisory Group for Neglected Tropical Diseases and an expert consultation agreed that the disease should no longer be considered endemic in the nine countries that had not reported any cases for decades. In the African Region these countries are Burundi, Cape Verde, Mauritius, Rwanda and the Seychelles; in the Region of the Americas they are Costa Rica, Suriname, and Trinidad and Tobago; and in the Western Pacific Region, the Solomon Islands. Following this decision, the number of countries requiring preventive chemotherapy was reduced from 81 to 72 (*1*) (*Fig. 3.14.1*).

Fig. 3.14.1 Global distribution and status of delivering preventive chemotherapy for lymphatic filariasis, 2010

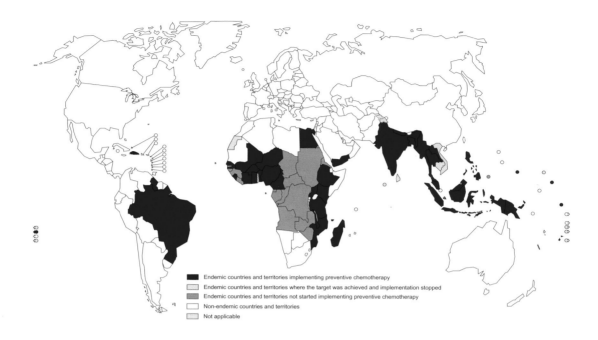

Endemic countries and territories implementing preventive chemotherapy
Endemic countries and territories where the target was achieved and implementation stopped
Endemic countries and territories not started implementing preventive chemotherapy
Non-endemic countries and territories
Not applicable

Impact

At least 40 million people have clinical manifestations of lymphatic filariasis
(*2*). Chronic disease causes acute dermatolymphangioadenitis, lymphoedema,
elephantiasis of limbs and hydrocele. These complications lead to impairment in
occupational activities, educational and employment opportunities, and mobility. The
disfigurement of limbs and genitals leads to stigma and discrimination. The impact
of eliminating lymphatic filariasis includes both social and economic benefits. These
benefits have been quantified at US$ 24 billion during 2000–2007 (*3*).

Strategy (roadmap targets and milestones)

In 2000, WHO established the Global Programme to Eliminate Lymphatic Filariasis
with the goal of eliminating the disease by 2020 (*4*). The programme has two strategic
goals. The first is to interrupt transmission and reduce the at-risk population to
zero. To achieve this goal, WHO recommended four sequential steps: (i) map the
geographical distribution of the disease; (ii) implement mass drug administration

annually for 5 years – with albendazole plus diethylcarbamazine, or in countries where onchocerciasis is endemic deliver albendazole plus ivermectin – to reduce the number of parasites in the blood to levels that will prevent mosquitoes from transmitting infection; (iii) initiate surveillance after mass drug administration has been discontinued; and (iv) verify that transmission has been eliminated (5).

The second goal is to provide access to a basic package of care to every affected person in endemic areas to manage complications and prevent disabilities. Simple hygiene measures can reduce the frequency of dermatolymphangioadenitis and improve lymphoedema, thus reducing progression to more advanced stages (elephantiasis). Surgery is recommended for hydrocele, and is offered in an increasing number of communities in endemic areas (2).

In 2011, WHO published new guidelines on how to evaluate the interruption of transmission and conduct surveillance after mass drug administration ceases by using transmission assessment surveys (5). WHO and its partners are also developing modules to train the staff of national programmes how to conduct the surveys.

Progress towards achieving the second goal (to provide a basic package of care) needs to be accelerated. Only about one third of national programmes have implemented morbidity management and disability prevention strategies for people with advanced cases of lymphatic filariasis. WHO is scaling up this component by producing guidelines, engaging in advocacy, systematically collecting data, and building capacity to develop adequate resources at international, national and local levels.

By 2010 the Global Programme to Eliminate Lymphatic Filariasis had reached the halfway point in its projected goal of eliminating the disease by 2020 (*Figs. 3.14.2–3.14.4*). Accordingly, a comprehensive review was carried out to assess the epidemiological situation of lymphatic filariasis and the progress that had been made towards elimination. The outcome of this review has been published (4). The milestones for the programme's strategic plan are: to ensure that by 2015 full geographical coverage with mass drug administration has been achieved in all endemic countries including those where loiasis and lymphatic filariasis are coendemic; and by 2020 ensure that 70% of countries have been verified as being free of lymphatic filariasis, with 30% engaging in postintervention surveillance.

Fig. 3.14.2 Projected scaling up and scaling down of the Global
Programme to Eliminate Lymphatic Filariasis, 2000–2020 (4)

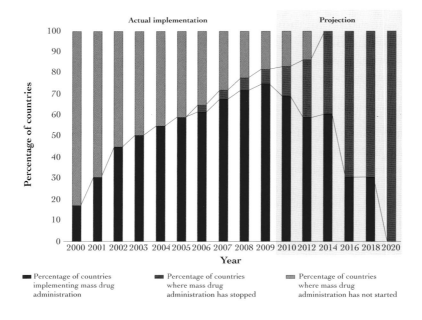

Fig. 3.14.3 Targets as the proportion of endemic countries expected to interrupt transmission in
the Global Programme to Eliminate Lymphatic Filariasis, by year, 2012–2020 (4)

Year	Category (objective)			
	Starting (implementation begun)	Scaling up MDA (full geographical coverage achieved)	Stopping interventions and starting surveillance (MDA stopped and post-MDA surveillance established)	Verifying absence of transmission (countries verified as free of lymphatic filariasis)
2012	85	70	25	20
2014	100	75	40	20
2016	100	100	70	40
2018	100	100	75	45
2020	100	100	100	70

MDA, mass drug administration
[a] Values are the proportion of country-based programmes that should achieve specified indicators for interrupting transmission.

DISEASES

Fig. 3.14.4 Milestones for the Global Programme to Eliminate Lymphatic Filariasis, 2010–2020 (4)

Year	Milestone
2011	• Revised WHO guidelines on interrupting transmission and conducting post-intervention surveillance completed and available
	• WHO guidelines and criteria for verifying absence of transmission completed and available
	• WHO guidelines and training modules for morbidity management completed and available
2012	• Mapping completed in all countries
	• MDA started in all countries without co-endemic loiasis
	• Provisional strategy for interrupting transmission in loiasis-endemic countries developed and circulated
	• 25% of endemic countries have met the criteria for stopping interventions and entered post-intervention surveillance phase
2013	• Revised strategy for interrupting transmission implemented in all loiasis-endemic countries
	• Metrics for annual reporting on morbidity-management programmes developed by WHO and disseminated
2014	• 20% of endemic countries verified free of transmission
	• All endemic countries collecting and reporting data on morbidity management to WHO
2015	• Full geographical coverage with MDA or other interventions, or both, achieved in all endemic urban areas
	• Full geographical coverage with MDA or other interventions, or both, achieved in all countries where loiasis is not endemic
	• Progress, global impact and remaining challenges assessed mid-plan
2016	• Full geographical coverage with MDA or other interventions, or both, achieved in countries with heaviest burden
	• Full geographical coverage with MDA or other interventions, or both, achieved in all countries with co-endemic loiasis
	• 70% of endemic countries have met the criteria for stopping interventions and entered into post-intervention surveillance phase
2020	• 70% of countries verified as free of lymphatic filariasis and 30% under post-intervention surveillance
	• Full geographical coverage and access to basic care for lymphoedema (and hydrocele in areas of bancroftian filariasis) offered in all countries

MDA, mass drug administration

REFERENCES

1   Global Programme to Eliminate Lymphatic Filariasis: progress report on mass drug administration, 2010. *Weekly Epidemiological Record*, 2011, 86:377–388.

2   *Managing morbidity and preventing disability in the Global Programme to Eliminate Lymphatic Filariasis: WHO position statement*. Geneva, World Health Organization, 2011 (WHO/HTM/NTD/PCT/2011.8).

3   Chu BK et al. The economic benefits resulting from the first 8 years of the Global Programme to Eliminate Lymphatic Filariasis (2000-2007). *PLoS Neglected Tropical Diseases*, 2012, 4:e708 (doi:10.1371/journal.pntd.0000708).

4   *Global Programme to Eliminate Lymphatic Filariasis: progress report 2000–2009 and strategic plan 2010–2020*. Geneva, World Health Organization, 2010 (WHO/HTM/NTD/PCT/2010.6).

5   *Monitoring and epidemiological assessment of mass drug administration: a manual for national elimination programmes*. Geneva, World Health Organization, 2011 (WHO/HTM/NTD/PCT/2011.4).

3.15   ONCHOCERCIASIS (RIVER BLINDNESS)

Introduction

Onchocerciasis is caused by infection with a filarial nematode (*Onchocerca volvulus*) transmitted by infected blackflies (*Simulium* spp.) that breed in fast-flowing rivers and streams. The adult worms produce embryonic microfilarial larvae that migrate to the skin, eyes and other organs (*1*).

Distribution

More than 99% of people infected with *O. volvulus* live in 30 sub-Saharan African countries, namely Angola, Benin, Burkina Faso, Burundi, Cameroon, the Central African Republic, Chad, Côte d'Ivoire, the Democratic Republic of the Congo, Equatorial Guinea, Ethiopia, Gabon, Ghana, Guinea, Guinea-Bissau, Kenya, Liberia, Malawi, Mali, Mozambique, Niger, Nigeria, Rwanda, Sierra Leone, Senegal, Sudan, South Sudan, Togo, Uganda and the United Republic of Tanzania. The infection also occurs in Yemen and six countries in Latin America (the Bolivarian Republic of Venezuela, Brazil, Colombia, Ecuador, Guatemala and Mexico). The distribution of onchocerciasis is shown in *Fig. 3.15.1*.

Fig. 3.15.1 Global distribution of onchocerciasis, 2011

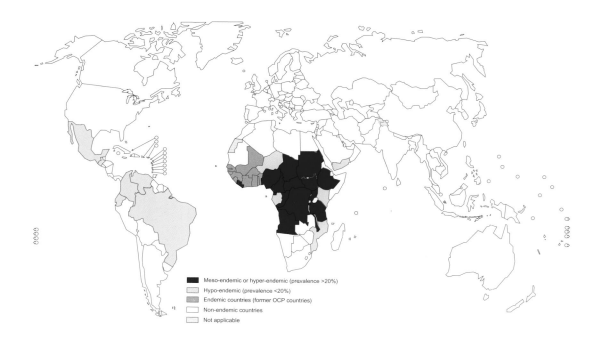

Meso-endemic or hyper-endemic (prevalence >20%)
Hypo-endemic (prevalence <20%)
Endemic countries (former OCP countries)
Non-endemic countries
Not applicable

Impact

The Onchocerciasis Control Programme in West Africa, which operated from 1974 to 2002, reduced levels of the infection and prevented eye lesions in 40 million people in 11 countries. About 600 000 cases of blindness were averted. In addition, 25 million hectares of abandoned arable land were reclaimed for settlement and agricultural production (2,3). The African Programme for Onchocerciasis Control started in 1995 and targets endemic countries that were not covered by the Onchocerciasis Control Programme (4).

The Onchocerciasis Elimination Program of the Americas was launched in 1992 in Latin America, and no cases of blindness attributable to the disease have been reported for more than 10 years – that is, since its launch.

Strategy (roadmap targets and milestones)

The Onchocerciasis Control Programme succeeded in eliminating onchocerciasis as a disease of public health importance and an obstacle to socioeconomic development in 10/11 endemic countries in West Africa, thereby reducing the prevalence of the disease below the threshold of 5%. The main interventions used were vector control and preventive chemotherapy with ivermectin. The decision was taken to continue regular surveillance and the delivery of preventive chemotherapy to safeguard the achievements of the programme (2,3).

The African Programme for Onchocerciasis Control has established programmes to deliver community-directed treatment with ivermectin and implement vector-control measures. It also provides preventive chemotherapy for other NTDs in areas where onchocerciasis is endemic (5,6).

The Onchocerciasis Elimination Programme of the Americas aims at eliminating ocular morbidity and interrupting transmission throughout the region by 2012. Good progress is being made in the region. All 13 foci achieved coverage of mass drug administration of more than 85% in 2006, and transmission had been interrupted in 10 foci by the end of 2011 (7).

A national action plan in Yemen aims at eliminating onchocerciasis by 2015 by delivering preventive chemotherapy with ivermectin, and implementing vector-control measures. However, political unrest has delayed implementation.

REFERENCES

[1] Crump A, Morel CM, Omura S. The onchocerciasis chronicle: from the beginning to the end? *Trends in Parasitology*, 2012, 28:280–288.

[2] *Ten years of onchocerciasis control in West Africa: review of the work of the Onchocerciasis Control Programme in the Volta River Basin area from 1974 to 1984*. Geneva, World Health Organization, 1985 (OCP/GVA/85).

[3] *Success in Africa: the Onchocerciasis Control Programme in West Africa 1974–2002*. Geneva, World Health Organization, 2002.

[4] Amazigo U et al. Onchocerciasis. In: Jamison DT et al, eds. *Disease and mortality in sub-Saharan Africa, 2nd ed*. Washington, DC, World Bank, 2006:1–11.

[5] Amazigo U. The African Programme for Onchocerciasis Control (APOC). *Annals of Tropical Medicine and Parasitology*, 2008, 102(Suppl.):S19–S22.

[6] African Programme for Onchocerciasis Control: meeting of national onchocerciasis task forces, September 2012. *Weekly Epidemiological Record*, 2012, 49/50:494–502.

[7] Progress towards eliminating onchocerciasis in the WHO Region of the Americas in 2011: interruption of transmission in Guatemala and Mexico, *Weekly Epidemiological Record*, 2012, 33:309–315.

DISEASES

3.16   SCHISTOSOMIASIS

Introduction

Schistosomiasis (also known as bilharzia) is a disease caused by infection with blood flukes of the genus *Schistosoma* (*1,2,3*) (*Table 3.16.1*). Most cases of disease result from infection with *S. haematobium* (which causes urogenital schistosomiasis) and *S. mansoni* (which causes intestinal schistosomiasis). Infected snails release larval stages of the organism (cercariae) into water. Human contact with water where the snails live is the source of the persistence of schistosomiasis.

Table 3.16.1 Type of schistosomiasis, *Schistosoma* species causing disease, distribution of species, and intermediate snail host

Type of schistosomiasis	*Schistosoma* species	Geographical distribution	Snail hosts
Intestinal schistosomiasis	S. mansoni	Africa, the Middle East, Caribbean islands, Brazil, Venezuela (Bolivirian Republic of), Suriname	*Biomphalaria* spp.
	S. japonicum	China, Indonesia, the Philippines	*Oncomelania* spp.
	S. mekongi	Cambodia and the Lao People's Democratic Republic	*Neotricula* spp.
	S. guineensis, S. intercalatum	Rainforest areas of central Africa	*Bulinus* spp.
Urogenital	S. haematobium	Africa, the Middle East	*Bulinus* spp.

Distribution

The distribution of schistosomiasis is focal, since transmission depends on specific snail hosts and human activities that lead to the contamination of water and infection. Schistosomiasis is endemic in five WHO regions (*Fig 3.16.1*).

Schistosomiasis has been reported from 78 countries, but no cases have been reported recently from 19 countries where transmission may have been interrupted (*4*). Estimates indicate that transmission is sufficiently intense to justify preventive chemotherapy in 52 countries. The status of transmission must be determined in the remaining 7 countries.

At least 237 million people need preventive chemotherapy for schistosomiasis; 90% of them live in sub-Saharan Africa (*5*). More than 70% of all cases live in 10 African countries (*Fig. 3.16.2*). In the Caribbean islands and Suriname, transmission is low and only a few or no cases have been detected in recent years; there is a need to

DISEASES

Fig. 3.16.1 Global distribution of schistosomiasis, 2011

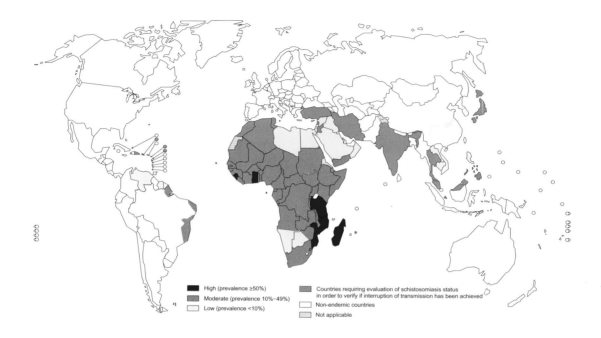

High (prevalence ≥50%)

Moderate (prevalence 10%–49%)

Low (prevalence <10%)

Countries requiring evaluation of schistosomiasis status
in order to verify if interruption of transmission has been achieved

Non-endemic countries

Not applicable

Fig. 3.16.2 Proportion of people requiring preventive chemotherapy for
schistosomiasis, by country, WHO African Region, 2010

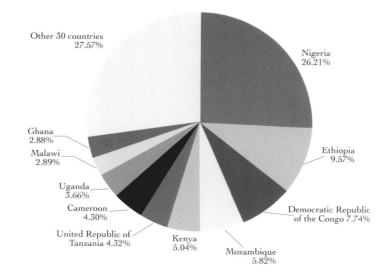

Other 30 countries
27.57%

Nigeria
26.21%

Ghana
2.88%

Malawi
2.89%

Uganda
3.66%

Cameroon
4.30%

United Republic of
Tanzania 4.32%

Kenya
5.04%

Mozambique
5.82%

Democratic Republic
of the Congo 7.74%

Ethiopia
9.57%

determine if elimination has been achieved. Low rates of transmission continue in Brazil and the Bolivarian Republic of Venezuela; transmission in many areas in these countries could be interrupted if control efforts were strengthened.

Control has been successful in the Eastern Mediterranean Region, where several countries need to determine whether transmission has been interrupted. Endemicity remains high in Somalia, Sudan and Yemen, although Yemen now has a strong national control programme.

In the Western Pacific Region, control of *S. japonicum* has been so successful that in China transmission will probably be interrupted by 2015 (*6*). Morbidity associated with *S. mekongi* has been controlled in Cambodia, but treatment campaigns will need to continue until strategies to prevent a resurgence of infection have been devised and a treatment programme has been launched in the neighbouring Lao People's Democratic Republic. High infection rates have been found in some provinces of the Philippines, and new endemic areas have been detected in Cagayan and Negros Occidental (*7*). Mass treatment campaigns were restarted in the Philippines in 2008 with the goal of achieving elimination.

Impact

Schistosomiasis is a serious chronic disease. Inflammatory immune responses to eggs trapped in tissues and organs result in pathology, anaemia, malnutrition, stunted growth, impaired cognitive development and reduced capacity to work (*1*). Intestinal schistosomiasis can progress from abdominal pain and bloody diarrhoea to hepatosplenomegaly, periportal liver fibrosis and portal hypertension. Urogenital schistosomiasis causes haematuria, dysuria and hydronephrosis, and can result in calcification of the bladder, and bladder cancer (*8*) as well as an increased risk of HIV infection (*9*).

Strategy (roadmap targets and milestones)

Treatment with praziquantel has been the mainstay of schistosomiasis control since 1984, and it has been used for preventive chemotherapy since 2006 (*10,11*). Many countries have implemented preventive chemotherapy programmes, and this has had beneficial impacts on morbidity, the prevalence of infection and transmission (*12,13,14*). In China, preventive chemotherapy was part of an integrated approach to control but it is now being used as part of an elimination strategy that focuses on controlling the source of infection (*6*). The progress made in delivering preventive chemotherapy with praziquantel in WHO's regions is shown in *Fig.3.16.3*. The goal of ensuring that at least 75% of school-aged children have access to preventive chemotherapy with praziquantel has still to be reached.

DISEASES

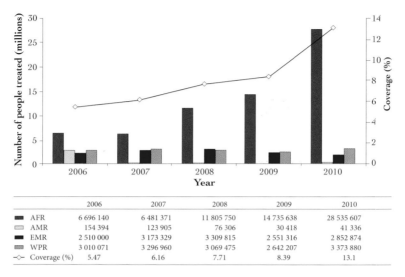

Fig. 3.16.3 Coverage of preventive chemotherapy and treatment for schistosomiasis, by WHO region, 2006–2010

	2006	2007	2008	2009	2010
■ AFR	6 696 140	6 481 371	11 805 750	14 735 638	28 535 607
▨ AMR	154 394	123 905	76 306	30 418	41 336
■ EMR	2 510 000	3 173 329	3 309 815	2 551 316	2 852 874
▨ WPR	3 010 071	3 296 960	3 069 475	2 642 207	3 373 880
◇ Coverage (%)	5.47	6.16	7.71	8.39	13.1

AFR – African Region / AMR–Region of the Americas / EMR–Eastern Mediterranean Region / WPR–Western Pacific Region

The plan for interrupting transmission and confirming elimination is outlined in *Table 3.16.2*. To effectively support the delivery of preventive chemotherapy, it is important to ensure that affected populations receive hygiene education, that sanitation is improved, that safe drinking-water is provided, and that snails are controlled.

The roadmap sets targets for control that also provide a means for assessing the implementation of control efforts. Schistosomiasis will be eliminated in the Caribbean, the Eastern Mediterranean Region, Indonesia and the Mekong River Basin by 2015. Interruption of transmission remains to be verified in 19 countries, including Algeria and Mauritius in the African Region.

The Sixty-fifth World Health Assembly adopted resolution WHA65.21 and this has been incorporated into the new strategic plan for schistosomiasis control (*Annex 1*). Additional targets have been set in the strategic plan; these will be used to assess progress during the next 9 years (*4*) (*Table 3.16.3*). The plan includes projections on the number of people who will be treated each year and the amount of praziquantel required through 2025 (*Fig. 3.16.4*). The number of people to be treated and the amount of praziquantel is projected to peak in 2018, at 235 million people and 645 million tablets. These estimates assume that all endemic countries will implement control programmes, and that transmission will be interrupted by some countries during the period covered by the plan.

Table 3.16.2 Goals, interventions, targets and timeline for making progress towards eliminating schistosomiasis

Group	Countries eligible for control of morbidity	Countries eligible for elimination as a public-health problem	Countries eligible for elimination (interruption of transmission)	V E R I F I C A T I O N	Countries that have achieved elimination
Goal	Control morbidity	Eliminate schistosomiasis as a public-health problem	Eliminate schistosomiasis (nterrupt transmission)		Implement post-elimination surveillance
Recommended interventions	Preventive chemotherapy Complementary public-health interventions where possible	Adjusted preventive chemotherapy Complementary public-health interventions strongly recommended	Intensified preventive chemotherapy in residual areas of transmission Complementary public-health interventions considered essential		Surveillance to detect and respond to resurgence of transmission and to prevent reintroduction
Targets	100% geographical coverage and ≥75% national coverage Prevalence of heavy-intensity infection <5% across sentinel sites	Prevalence of heavy-intensity infection <1% in all sentinel sites	Reduce incidence of infection to zero		Incidence of infection remains zero (no cases)
Estimated time to progress from one group to the next	Up to 5–10 years from joining the group	Up to 3–6 years from joining the group	Up to 5 years from joining the group		To continue until all countries have interrupted transmission

Fig. 3.16.4   Percentage of countries implementing preventive chemotherapy for schistosomiasis of those where it is required, 2008–2020

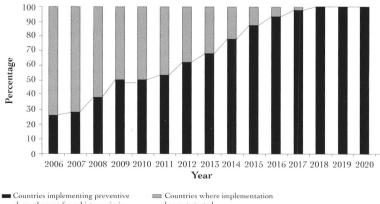

■ Countries implementing preventive chemotherapy for schistosomiasis   ▨ Countries where implementation has not started

DISEASES

Table 3.16.3 Targets and milestones for eliminating schistosomiasis

Year	Milestones
2012	• Global strategic plan for schistosomiasis adopted
	• Global coordination mechanism put in place to ensure
	– adequate supply of praziquantel
	– resources for country-level implementation
	– harmonization of partners' activities
	• National policies for controlling NTDs, including schistosomiasis, in place in 50% of the countries requiring preventive chemotherapy
	• A manual for schools about deworming including monitoring and evaluation published
	• Resolution on schistosomiasis elimination adopted by World Health Assembly
2013	• National plans of action for NTD control are developed by 75% of countries requiring preventive chemotherapy for schistosomiasis
	• Procedures and guidelines for verifying interruption of transmission are established
	• Interruption of transmission is verified in countries that request it
	• Geographical mapping of ≥75% of countries requiring preventive chemotherapy is completed, and WHO's Preventive Chemotherapy and Transmission Control Databank is updated
	• Guidelines for snail control are revised and disseminated
	• Training is conducted for NTD programme managers
	• Standard operating procedures to monitor the efficacy of praziquantel are developed
2015	• Multisectoral approach to NTDs is addressed in all national plans of action; sectors addressed include water and sanitation, education and agriculture
	• National plans of action for NTDs, including schistosomiasis, are adopted in all endemic countries
	• 100% geographical coverage of preventive chemotherapy and ≥75% national coverage is reached in ≥50% of the countries requiring preventive chemotherapy
	• A standardized system to monitor the efficacy of large-scale use of praziquantel is designed and put in place
2016	• Mid-term evaluation of the Strategic Plan is completed
2019	• Preparation of the Strategic Plan for 2020 and beyond is finalized
2020	• ≥75% national coverage is reached in all the countries requiring preventive chemotherapy for schistosomiasis

NTD, neglected tropical disease

REFERENCES

[1] Gryseels B. Schistosomiasis. *Infectious Disease Clinics of North America*, 2012, 26:383–397.

[2] Shiff C. The importance of definitive diagnosis in chronic schistosomiasis, with reference to *Schistosoma haematobium*. *Journal . Research*, 2012, 2012:761269 (doi: 10.1155/2012/761269).

[3] Silva LC et al. Ultrasound and magnetic resonance imaging findings in *Schistosomiasis mansoni*: expanded gallbladder fossa and fatty hilum signs. *Revista da Sociedade Brasileira de Medicina Tropical*, 2012, 45:500–504.

[4] *Schistosomiasis: progress report 2001–2011 and strategic plan 2012–2020*. Geneva, World Health Organization, 2012 (WHO/HTM/NTD/2012.7).

5   Schistosomiasis: population requiring preventive chemotherapy and number of people treated in 2010. *Weekly Epidemiological Record*, 2012, 87:37–44.

6   Wang LD et al. A strategy to control transmission of *Schistosoma japonicum* in China. *New England Journal of Medicine*, 2009, 360:121–128.

7   Leonardo L et al. A national baseline prevalence survey of schistosomiasis in the Philippines using stratified two-step systematic cluster sampling design. *Journal of Tropical Medicine*, 2012, 2012:936128 (doi:10.1155/2012/936128).

8   Parkin DM. The global burden of urinary bladder cancer. *Scandinavian Journal of Urology and Nephrology*, 2008, 42(Suppl. 218):S12–S20.

9   Kjetland EF et al. Association between genital schistosomiasis and HIV in rural Zimbabwean women. *AIDS*, 2006, 20:593–600.

10 *The control of schistosomiasis: report of a WHO expert committee*. Geneva, World Health Organization, 1985 (WHO Technical Report Series, No. 728).

11 *Preventive chemotherapy in human helminthiasis*. Geneva, World Health Organization, 2006.

12 Utzinger J et al. Conquering schistosomiasis in China: the long march. *Acta Tropica*, 2005, 96:69–96.

13 Kabatereine NB et al. Impact of a national helminth control programme on infection and morbidity in Ugandan schoolchildren. *Bulletin of the World Health Organization*, 2007, 85:91–99.

14 Touré S et al. Two-year impact of single praziquantel treatment on infection in the national control programme on schistosomiasis in Burkina Faso. *Bulletin of the World Health Organization*, 2008, 86:780–787.

3.17   SOIL-TRANSMITTED HELMINTHIASES

Introduction

The most common nematode species that cause soil-transmitted helminthiases are *Ascaris lumbricoides*, *Trichuris trichiura*, *Necator americanus* and *Ancylostoma duodenale* (*1–3*). Morbidity can be controlled by delivering preventive chemotherapy with anthelminthic medicines; elimination and eradication will not be achieved until affected populations have access to effective sanitation, and sewage treatment and disposal.

Distribution

WHO estimates that about 890 million children require annual treatment with preventive chemotherapy (*4*). The global distribution of soil-transmitted helminthiases is shown in *Fig.3.17*.1 as is the proportion of children who need regular preventive chemotherapy. The proportion of children needing treatment, by country, in 2010 is shown in *Fig.3.17.2*.

Fig. 3.17.1 Distribution of soil-transmitted helminthiases and proportion of children (aged 1–14 years) in each endemic country requiring preventive chemotherapy for the diseases, 2011

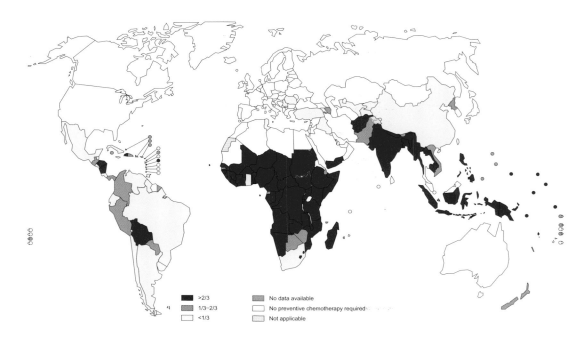

■ >2/3	▨ No data available
▨ 1/3–2/3	□ No preventive chemotherapy required
□ <1/3	▨ Not applicable

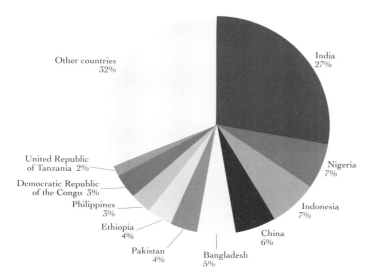

Fig. 3.17.2 Proportion of children requiring preventive chemotherapy for soil-transmitted helminthiases, by country, 2010

India 27%
Nigeria 7%
Indonesia 7%
China 6%
Bangladesh 5%
Pakistan 4%
Ethiopia 4%
Philippines 3%
Democratic Republic of the Congo 3%
United Republic of Tanzania 2%
Other countries 32%

Impact

At the beginning of the 20th century, the Rockefeller Foundation was the first to promote regular deworming as a successful public-health intervention for reducing absenteeism from school and work. This finding has been supported by more recent evaluations showing that school-based mass deworming programmes reduced absenteeism (5), and increased adults' earnings (6) in Kenya.

The Cochrane Database of Systemic Reviews (7) concluded that screening children for intestinal helminths and then treating infected children appears to be a promising intervention, but the evidence is slight. However, the review also found that treating children for soil-transmitted helminthiases improved their nutritional status, school attendance and learning. The review should serve as a reminder of the need to continue evaluating programmes that treat school-aged children for helminth infections. WHO will review recent findings about the impact of deworming and revise its guidelines if necessary.

At this stage, however, three other aspects of the deworming intervention should be considered. First, parents, caregivers and teachers in many communities approve of these programmes and show excellent compliance with the treatments. Secondly, each year children die from intestinal obstructions or endure other complications from these infections, some of which require surgical intervention that is not always available (8,9). Thirdly, there is a moral dimension. If it is known that many children are infected, should they not have access to regular treatment with quality-assured medicines? If screening to detect infection is added to current interventions, these programmes will become too expensive for all but a few places where these infections are prevalent.

Strategy (roadmap targets and milestones)

The strategic plan for eliminating soil-transmitted helminthiases as a public-health problem in children (*10*) set five milestones for 2012, and all have been reached (*Table 3.17.1*).

The main intervention recommended by WHO for controlling soil-transmitted helminthiases is to regularly administer preventive chemotherapy with albendazole or mebendazole. Global coverage of the medicines used to prevent these infections

Table 3.17.1 Milestones for eliminating soil-transmitted helminthiases as a public-health problem in children

Year	Milestone
2012	• Communication strategy for control of STH (and other NTDs) developed
	• Regional programme review groups expanded
	• National plans of action for NTD control developed by 50% of countries requiring preventive chemotherapy for STH
	• National policies for STH control involving intersectoral collaboration (for example, from education and water and sanitation sectors) exist in 50% of countries requiring preventive chemotherapy for STH
	• Standard operating procedures to evaluate drug resistance developed
2013	• National plans of action for NTD control developed by 75% of countries requiring preventive chemotherapy for STH
	• National policies for STH control involving intersectoral collaboration (for example, in education and water and sanitation sectors) exist in 75% of countries requiring preventive chemotherapy for STH
	• Manuals for control of STH in all at-risk groups produced and disseminated
	• Mapping to identify areas requiring preventive chemotherapy completed in all countries where STH are endemic
2015	• National plans of action for NTD control developed by 100% of countries requiring preventive chemotherapy for STH
	• National policies for STH control involving intersectoral collaboration (for example, in education and water and sanitation sectors) available in 100% of countries requiring preventive chemotherapy for STH
	• 50% of countries requiring preventive chemotherapy for STH have achieved 75% national coverage of SAC and pre-SAC, and 50% of SAC and pre-SAC needing treatment worldwide have been treated
2020	• 100% of countries requiring preventive chemotherapy for STH have achieved 75% national coverage of SAC and pre-SAC
	• 100% of countries requiring preventive chemotherapy for STH regularly assess intensity of the infections in sentinel sites
	• Less than 1% of countries requiring preventive chemotherapy for STH have infection of high or moderate intensity
	• 75–100% of children (SAC and pre-SAC) needing preventive chemotherapy worldwide have been treated

NTD, neglected tropical disease; pre-SAC, preschool-age children; SAC, school-age children; STH, soil-transmitted helminthiases increased significantly during 2009, reaching more than 273 million children or roughly 30% of those in need. In 2010, this number remained constant (*4*). The coverage of deworming treatments delivered to children from 2006 to 2010 is shown in *Fig.3.17.3*.

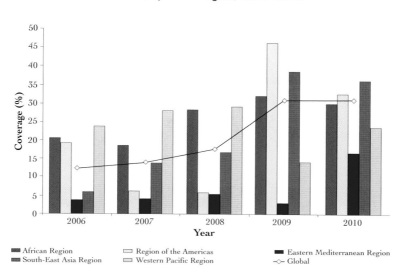

Fig. 3.17.3   Reported coverage of treatment (%) for soil-transmitted helminthiases, by WHO region, 2006–2010

Coverage was scaled up significantly during 2011–2012. Beginning in 2012, 600 million tablets of albendazole or mebendazole became available annually to treat school-aged children in endemic countries. Although complete coverage data for 2011–2012 are not yet available, countries have requested an additional 150 million tablets, indicating a significant increase in coverage. The number of tablets expected to be required annually to treat all school-aged and preschool-aged children who need treatment from now until 2020 is shown in *Fig.3.17.4*.

WHO released two publications to support the scaling up of helminthiases-control efforts that target children (*11,12*). Applying this guidance will help national programmes managers to achieve the milestones set by WHO in the roadmap (*13*) and in the strategic plan 2011–2020 (*10*).

DISEASES

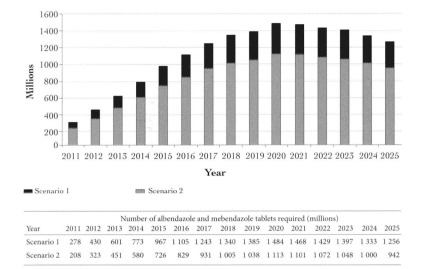

Fig. 3.17.4 Projected number of anthelminthics medicines required to achieve the global targets for treating preschool-aged and school-aged children, 2020–2025 (*11*)

Number of albendazole and mebendazole tablets required (millions)															
Year	2011	2012	2013	2014	2015	2016	2017	2018	2019	2020	2021	2022	2023	2024	2025
Scenario 1	278	430	601	773	967	1 105	1 243	1 340	1 385	1 484	1 468	1 429	1 397	1 333	1 256
Scenario 2	208	323	451	580	726	829	931	1 005	1 038	1 113	1 101	1 072	1 048	1 000	942

Scenario 1: All countries reach 100% national coverage by 2020
Scenario 2: All countries reach 75% national coverage by 2020

REFERENCES

1   Hall A et al. A review and meta-analysis of the impact of intestinal worms on child growth and nutrition. *Maternal and Child Nutrition*, 2008, 4(Suppl. 1):S118–S236.

2   Nokes C et al. Parasitic helminth infection and cognitive function in school children. *Proceedings of the Royal Society of London B*, 1992, 247:77–81.

3   Crompton DWT, Nesheim MC. Nutritional impact of intestinal helminthiasis during the human life cycle. *Annual Review of Nutrition*, 2002, 22:35–59.

4   Soil-transmitted helminthiases: number of children treated in 2010. *Weekly Epidemiological Record*, 2012, 87:225–232.

5   Miguel M, Kramer M. Worms: identifying impacts on education and health in the presence of treatment externalities. *Econometrica*, 2004, 72:159–217.

6   Bleakley H. Diseases and development: evidence for hookworm eradication in the American south. Report of the Rockefeller Sanitary Commission. *Quarterly Journal of Economics*, 2007, 122:73–117.

7   Taylor-Robinson DC et al. Deworming drugs for soil-transmitted intestinal worms in children: effects on nutritional indicators, haemoglobin and school performance. *Cochrane Database of Systematic Reviews*, 2007(4):CD000371 (doi: 10.1002/14651858.CD000371.pub3).

8   de Silva NR, Chan MS, Bundy DA. Morbidity and mortality due to ascariasis: re-estimation and sensitivity analysis of global numbers at risk. *Tropical Medicine and International Health*, 1997, 2:519–528.

9   Wani I et al. Intestinal ascariasis in children. *World Journal of Surgery*, 2010, 34:963–938.

10   *Eliminating soil-transmitted helminthiases as a public health problem in children: progress report 2001–2010 and strategic plan 2011–2020*. Geneva, World Health Organization, 2012 (WHO/HTM/NTD/PCT/2012.4).

11   *Assuring the safety of preventive chemotherapy for the control of neglected diseases*. Geneva, World Health Organization, 2011.

12   *Helminth control in school-age children: a guide for managers of control programmes, 2nd ed*. Geneva, World Health Organization, 2011.

13   *Accelerating work to overcome the global impact of neglected tropical diseases: a roadmap for implementation*. Geneva, World Health Organization, 2012 (WHO/HTM/NTD/2012.1).

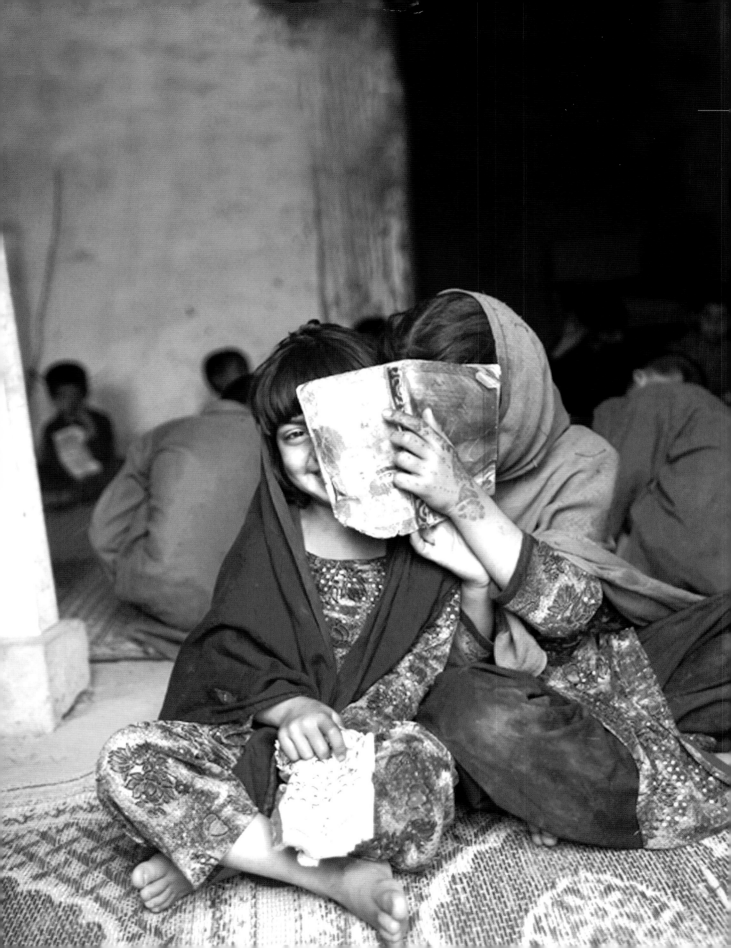

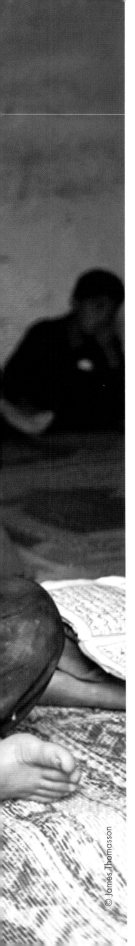

© James Thomasson

KEY INTERVENTIONS: SITUATION REPORT

WHO promotes the use of five public-health strategies to control, eliminate and eradicate NTDs; these provide (i) preventive chemotherapy; (ii) innovative and intensified disease-management; (iii) vector control and pesticide management; (iv) safe drinking-water, basic sanitation and hygiene services, and education; (v) and veterinary public-health services using the one-health concept.

WHO promotes the use of five public-health strategies to control, eliminate and eradicate NTDs; these provide (i) preventive chemotherapy; (ii) innovative and intensified disease-management; (iii) vector control and pesticide management; (iv) safe drinking-water, basic sanitation and hygiene services, and education; (v) and veterinary public-health services using the one-health concept. Each strategy requires implementation of a group of activities. For example, delivering preventive chemotherapy includes providing information and education to the target community, training health workers, using epidemiological information to ensure appropriate and timely access to quality-assured medicines, engaging in pharmacovigilance, ensuring that procedures used to deliver medicines are safe, accurately monitoring treatment coverage, evaluating outcomes, and providing feedback to the community about the process and outcomes of the intervention. Equivalent numbers of components exist for the other strategies. A combination of public-health strategies will be needed to achieve control of each NTD. For example, human African trypanosomiasis will not be overcome without continued and regular surveillance of endemic foci, vector-control measures and intensified case-management that includes ensuring people have access to prompt and accurate diagnosis, and medical attention.

4.1   PREVENTIVE CHEMOTHERAPY

As a public-health strategy, preventive chemotherapy aims to reduce the burden of disease. In the context of NTDs, preventive chemotherapy is defined as the widespread delivery of safe, single-dose, quality-assured medicines, either alone or in combination, at regular intervals to treat selected diseases (*1*). Preventive chemotherapy is recommended by WHO as a public-health intervention for lymphatic filariasis, onchocerciasis, schistosomiasis, soil-transmitted helminthiases and blinding trachoma. Preventive chemotherapy is a component of the established SAFE strategy for trachoma (Surgery, Antibiotics, Facial cleanliness and Environmental improvements). Preventive chemotherapy is also helpful in controlling morbidity from some foodborne trematodiases (see *section 3.13*).

Other supportive interventions include providing management for chronic cases and people with disabilities, controlling vectors and intermediate hosts, providing veterinary public-health services, and providing safe drinking-water, and sanitation and hygiene services. Implementing preventive chemotherapy and attaining high coverage should ensure that by 2020 WHO's goals will have been reached for lymphatic filariasis, onchocerciasis, schistosomiasis, soil-transmitted helminthiases and trachoma, and that some regional and subregional milestones will be reached by 2015 (*2*).

In areas where preventive chemotherapy is recommended for more than one disease, integrating and coordinating activities for all relevant diseases, including strategic and operational planning, is as important as for a programme targeting a single disease. Decisions about integrating activities should be based on optimization criteria, which include cost-effectiveness, the ability to enhance impacts, political advantages, logistical convenience, timing and safety. For programmes to run efficiently, they must be cost effective, raise the visibility of NTDs, and the interventions must be acceptable to the affected population.

The number of countries eligible for preventive chemotherapy and the types of infections transmitted in each country are shown in *Fig. 4.1.1*. Of the 123 countries requiring preventive chemotherapy, 40 require interventions for three or more diseases; 33 of the 40 are in the African Region. Implementing an integrated approach to disease control and elimination is strongly indicated in high-burden countries.

Since the release of the first report on NTDs in 2010, global efforts have been accelerated to scale up integrated and coordinated planning to deliver preventive chemotherapy. Disease-specific global and regional plans, and policies, guidelines and manuals have been published to assist Member States, and their donors and partners. Programmatic tools to facilitate integrated planning for and reporting on the delivery of preventive chemotherapy – such as a joint request for medicines

KEY INTERVENTIONS: SITUATION REPORT

Fig. 4.1.1   Countries requiring preventive chemotherapy for at least one neglected tropical disease (lymphatic filariasis, onchocerciaasiss, schistosmiasis or soil-transmitted helminthiases) and number of those diseases in each country, 2011

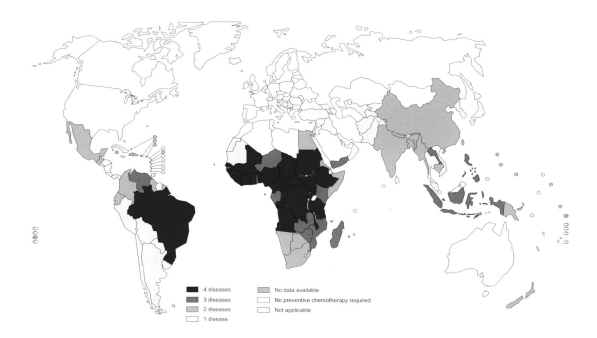

for preventive chemotherapy, the joint reporting form and the tool for integrated planning and costing – have been refined. Training modules have been developed, and regional and subregional workshops have been organized to help programme managers build their capacity to plan strategies, implement interventions, and monitor and evaluate outcomes.

Estimates of the number of people who require preventive chemotherapy have been revised for each disease, based on the most recent epidemiological and demographic information. Analyses have been carried out to determine the geographical overlap of the different diseases targeted by chemotherapy and the number of people requiring at least one intervention. About 1.9 billion people in 123 countries require preventive chemotherapy for at least one NTD; 55% of them require preventive treatment for one or two diseases, and 45% require it for three or more diseases (*Table 4.1.1*). (Since South Sudan became independent in 2011, the number of countries where preventive chemotherapy is needed has risen to 124.)

These analyses do not include the number of people with trachoma who need treatment with azithromycin. However, data reported for 2010 show that there are about 38.5 million active trachoma cases worldwide, and about 95% of these are in the African Region (*5*). It is unlikely that the number of people who need treatment for trachoma would substantially increase the total population already requiring an intervention for at least one disease annually.

Table 4.1.1 Estimated number of people requiring preventive chemotherapy by disease, and total number of people requiring preventive chemotherapy for at least one disease, by WHO region in 2010

WHO region	No. of people requiring preventive chemotherapy (millions)				Total no. of people requiring preventive chemotherapy (millions) for at least one disease
	Lymphatic filariasis	Soil-transmitted helminthiases	Schistosomiasis	Onchocerciasis	
African	431.8	290.1	220.6	116.4	597.7
Americas	11.8	45.3	1.5	0.5	54
South-East Asia	883.7	371.6	0	NA	1 014.7
Eastern Mediterranean	23.9	79.2	14.5	6.4	102.2
European	NA	4.3	NA	NA	4.3
Western Pacific	4.7	99.3	0.6	NA	128.7
All regions	1 355.9	889.8	237.2	123.3	1 901.6

NA, not applicable.

⁰ The total number of people requiring preventive chemotherapy for schistosomiasis in the South-East Asia Region is 2937.

In 2010, approximately 711 million people received preventive chemotherapy for at least one disease: 484 million for lymphatic filariasis, 330 million for soil-transmitted helminthiases, 81 million for onchocerciasis, and 35 million for schistosomiasis (*Table 4.1.2*). Data reported on treatment for trachoma show that 38.5 million people received antibiotics in 2010 (*3*).

The number of people treated for schistosomiasis almost tripled between 2005 and 2010, entirely due to the scaling up of programmes in the African Region. Similarly, the coverage for soil-transmitted helminthiases significantly increased between 2005 and 2010, reaching 31% of those considered to be at risk in 2010. By the end of 2010, mass drug administration for lymphatic filariasis had been implemented in 53 countries; 12 of these countries had implemented five or more rounds of preventive chemotherapy and achieved a prevalence of microfilaraemia of less than 1%, which enabled them to move to the surveillance stage of the elimination process. Onchocerciasis control programmes achieved their target of 65% coverage in 2010.

Of the 711 million people reached with preventive chemotherapy in 2010, almost half of them (355 million) live in Bangladesh and India, and received preventive treatment for lymphatic filariasis or soil-transmitted helminthiases, or both. Large parts of Bangladesh and India, and other countries, will meet the criteria for stopping preventive chemotherapy for lymphatic filariasis by 2015 and move towards surveillance, leading to a substantial decrease in the number of people

KEY INTERVENTIONS: SITUATION REPORT

Table 4.1.2 Number of people who received preventive chemotherapy, and number of people covered by preventive chemotherapy for at least 1 disease, by WHO region, 2010

WHO region	No. of countries reporting	No. of people requiring preventive chemotherapy				Total no. of people requiring preventive chemotherapy for at least one disease
		Lymphatic filariasis	Soil-transmitted helminthiases	Schistosomiasis	Onchocerciasis	
African	37	82 800 490	98 773 129	28 758 482	77 394 184	195 382 326
Americas	13	4 144 720	43 133 670	41 336	312 210	46 193 031
South-East Asia	7	380 402 738	144 509 399	ND	NA	409 558 865
Eastern Mediterranean	7	496 292	14 748 128	2 852 874	3 311 208	19 591 651
European	3	NA	1 386 539	NA	NA	1 386 539
Western Pacific	11	15 896 746	27 225 908	3 373 880	NA	39 024 779
Global	78	483 740 986	329 776 773	35 026 572	81 017 602	711 140 531
% at risk reached		35	31	13	66	37

NA, not applicable; ND, no data available

worldwide who are estimated to need preventive chemotherapy. Sustained progress in delivering preventive chemotherapy for lymphatic filariasis through mass drug administration has been possible because programmes have been able to take advantage of existing infrastructure. This infrastructure can be used by countries to transition to other disease-control interventions, especially those to control soil-transmitted helminthiases. If other control measures are not implemented, the gains made by delivering preventive chemotherapy will not be sustained.

Global coverage with preventive chemotherapy should expand significantly in the next few years as result of (i) the increased availability of donated medicines, (ii) the development of national action plans for delivering integrated preventive chemotherapy in all WHO regions, and (iii) the commitments to strengthen efforts to overcome NTDs made by national governments and supported by growing interest from donor agencies. However, by the end of 2010, only 25 countries or territories had achieved at least one of the targets set for delivering preventive chemotherapy for lymphatic filariasis, onchocerciasis or soil-transmitted helminthiases. Only five of these countries had reached their targets for delivering preventive chemotherapy for three or more diseases simultaneously. Therefore, interventions will need to be scaled up considerably if targets set in the World Health Assembly's resolutions are to be met (*Annex 1*).

Fig. 4.1.2 shows the percentage of people who require preventive chemotherapy together with a projection of the percentage that will need preventive chemotherapy if the roadmap's targets are to be met. Programmes must be scaled up faster.

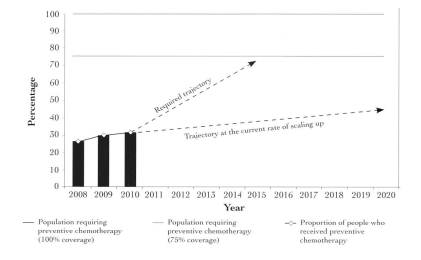

Fig. 4.1.2   Percentage of global population receiving preventive chemotherapy for at least one neglected tropical disease (lymphatic filariasis, schistosomiasis or soil-transmitted helminthiases) of the estimated population who need preventive chemotherapy (excluding India and Bangladesh), 2008–2020

— Population requiring preventive chemotherapy (100% coverage)

— Population requiring preventive chemotherapy (75% coverage)

–◇– Proportion of people who received preventive chemotherapy

REFERENCES

[1]   *Preventive chemotherapy in human helminthiasis. Coordinated use of anthelminthic drugs in control interventions: a manual for health professionals and programme managers,* Geneva, World Health Organization, 2012.

[2]   *Accelerating work to overcome the global impact of neglected tropical diseases: a roadmap for implementation.* Geneva, World Health Organization, 2012 (WHO/HTM/NTD/2012.1).

[3]   Global WHO Alliance for the Elimination of Blinding Trachoma by 2020. *Weekly Epidemiological Record,* 2012, 87:161–168.

4.2 INNOVATIVE AND INTENSIFIED DISEASE-MANAGEMENT

Innovative and intensified disease-management focuses on NTDs that are difficult to diagnose and treat, and can, in most cases, trigger severe clinical manifestations and complications. These are Buruli ulcer, Chagas disease, both forms of human African trypanosomiasis, the Leishmaniases (cutaneous, mucocutaneous and visceral forms), leprosy and yaws. Treatment for these diseases requires individual case-management, and there are few preventive measures that can be implemented on a large scale.

Given the complexity of these diseases, patients need to be seen at well equipped hospitals and by well trained, specialized technicians. Systematic screening of exposed populations is necessary because these diseases are generally asymptomatic during the period when treatments would be more effective and have less dangerous side-effects. The key aims of case management are to (i) diagnose cases early, (ii) provide treatment to cure or reduce infection and morbidity, (iii) manage complications, and (iv) adopt strategies to respond appropriately to different levels of endemicity and health-system capacity.

Four main approaches are recommended to prevent and control these NTDs.

- **Intensified control**. This approach seeks to ensure early diagnosis, prompt treatment, available and affordable medicines, properly equipped treatment centres, high-quality care, systematic screening, and appropriate monitoring and epidemiological surveillance.
- **Innovation**. This approach includes implementing strategies adapted to the capacities of national health systems and the epidemiology of the diseases, and, where necessary, modifying interventions.
- **Research and development**. This approach seeks to provide new diagnostics and safer medicines that can be used in remote and otherwise difficult settings.
- **Capacity strengthening**. This approach includes efforts to maintain and generate needed expertise at the national level and to improve programmes' abilities to adapt to local conditions.

A major contribution to expanding innovation and intensified disease-management in 2011 was the signing of an agreement for the donation of liposomal amphotericin B for control efforts targeting visceral Leishmaniasis (*Annex 2*). The distribution of the medicines will be supported by a grant from the United Kingdom's Department for International Development that will be used to enable capacity strengthening and provide logistical support to treat the disease in several endemic countries.

4.3   VECTOR CONTROL

The Vector Ecology and Management unit of WHO's Department of Control of Neglected Tropical Diseases promotes vector control through integrated vector management (VEM) and sound management of public-health pesticides. The unit houses WHOPES (the WHO Pesticide Evaluation Scheme), an international programme that coordinates the testing and evaluation of pesticides for use in public health and acts as the focal point within WHO for public-health pesticide management.

The unit advocates the IVM approach, defined as a rational decision-making process for the optimal use of resources (1), which is a component of WHO's Global plan to combat neglected tropical diseases (2). The IVM approach incorporates the application of sound ecological principles to reduce vectorial capacity, and it can be used against single or multiple vector-borne diseases simultaneously. IVM also offers immense opportunities for integrating control efforts among programmes.

To assist vector control programmes in countries endemic for or at risk of vector-borne diseases and to develop and adopt IVM, the unit has published four guiding documents: a guidance on policy-making (3), a core structure for training curricula (4), a handbook on IVM (5), and indicators for monitoring and evaluation of IVM (6). A WHO regional course on IVM was organized in WHO's South-East Asia Region in 2011. The unit works in collaboration with the preventive chemotherapy unit and the WHO Global Malaria Programme to promote a multiple disease control IVM approach in areas endemic for lymphatic filariasis, loaisis and malaria and to achieve elimination of lymphatic filariasis in areas endemic for *Loa loa*. The unit will continue to advocate implementation of sustainable vector control activities based on the principles of IVM and through strong multi-stakeholder and multi-sectoral approaches.

The use of insecticides has increased significantly in recent years due to an intensified focus on and investment in controlling vector-borne diseases (7,8). In 2010, a WHO survey in 142 countries found that the regulation of pesticides for public-health use by Member States was generally inadequate, that Member States lacked comprehensive pesticide legislation, that there was inadequate coordination in the registration of public-health pesticides, that Member States lacked published guidelines for registering public-health pesticides, and that there was inadequate compliance with and enforcement of regulations in the health sector (9,10). Additionally, the survey also found that a high proportion of pesticides sold were substandard, illegal or counterfeit, and that Member States were unable to provide adequate quality control for pesticides. Member States also lacked the capacity to safely dispose of pesticide containers and pesticide-related waste. On the positive side, 62% of countries have adopted the IVM policy for controlling vector-borne diseases; and 90% of countries reported including WHO's specifications for quality control in their requirements for pesticide procurement. Altogether, 74% required that WHOPES recommendations be followed for national registration of public-health pesticides (*11*).

The collaboration between WHO and FAO to provide unified, coordinated and consistent support to Member States and other stakeholders on the sound management of pesticides has been strengthened. This collaboration has included publication of guidelines on the registration and quality control of pesticides, and publication of WHO specifications for six pesticide products.

Since publication of the first WHO report on NTDs in 2010, WHOPES has also published peer-reviewed guidelines on procuring pesticides for public-health use (*12*), monitoring the durability of long-lasting insecticidal nets (*13*), testing the efficacy of insecticide products used to disinfect aircraft (*14*), and developing risk assessment models for different uses of pesticides (*15–17*). During the past 2 years, WHOPES has supported more than 20 Member States in conducting situation analyses and needs assessments for the use of pesticides, and has assisted four WHO regions (African, Americas, Eastern Mediterranean and South-East Asia) in developing regional policies and frameworks for pesticide management. During 2010–2012, WHOPES finalized its evaluation of, and made recommendations on, eight pesticide products for use in public health; another 18 pesticides are undergoing evaluation (*18*).

The dwindling arsenal of insecticides calls for the development of safe and effective products for vector control, and reducing as much as possible the time needed to bring new products to market. In collaboration with the Global Malaria Programme, the unit has established the Vector Control Advisory Group on New Tools to support the assessment of new technologies and approaches to controlling vector-borne diseases. The constitutional structure and procedures of this body are designed to ensure its transparency, independence and technical quality, and to ensure there is dialogue with external stakeholders as well as technical input from industry.

The WHO public–private partnership – Global Collaboration on Development of Pesticides for Public Health (GCDPP) – established in 1997, has been used in promoting the urgent need for development of alternative insecticides and application technologies, as well as strengthening collaboration with major stakeholders, including pesticide industry, as major partners in sound management of pesticides. The theme of the eighth GCDPP Meeting (held at WHO headquarters in Geneva on 20–21 February 2012) was dengue surveillance and vector management.

To ensure that the full potential of vector control is used to control the transmission of vector-borne NTDs, countries must strengthen their capacities in medical entomology, entomological surveillance, and operational research. The lack of a career path for entomologists has nurtured a migration towards academic research and away from public-health entomology. This trend needs to be reversed. When countries consider developing human capacity, attention must be paid to the skills required for effective programme management, including financing, logistics and promotional activity. The unit will continue to play a key part in developing appropriate training tools and courses in vector control and pesticide management.

REFERENCES

[1] *Global strategic framework for integrated vector management*. Geneva, World Health Organization, 2004 (WHO/CDS/CPE/PVC/2004.10).

[2] *Global plan to combat neglected tropical diseases 2008–2015*. Geneva, World Health Organization, 2007 (WHO/CDS/NTD/2007.3).

[3] van den Berg H, Mutero CM, Ichimori K. *Guidance on policy-making for integrated vector management*. Geneva, World Health Organization, 2012 (WHO/HTM/NTD/VEM/2012.2).

[4] *Core structure for training curricula on integrated vector management*. Geneva, World Health Organization, 2012 (WHO/HTM/NTD/VEM/2012.1).

[5] *Handbook for integrated vector management*. Geneva, World Health Organization, 2012 (WHO/HTM/NTD/VEM/2012.3).

[6] *Monitoring and evaluation indicators for integrated vector management*. Geneva, World Health Organization, 2012.

[7] van den Berg H et al. Global trends in the use of insecticides to control vector-borne diseases. *Environmental Health Perspectives*, 2012, 120:577–582 (doi:10.1289/ehp.1104340).

[8] *Global insecticide use for vector-borne disease control: a 10-year assessment, 2000–2009, 5th ed*. Geneva, World Health Organization, 2011 (WHO/HTM/NTD/VEM/WHOPES/2011.6).

[9] *Public health pesticide registration and management practices by WHO Member States: report of a survey, 2010*. Geneva, World Health Organization; 2011 (WHO/HTM/NTD/WHOPES/2010).

[10] Matthews GM et al. Status of legislation and regulatory control of public health pesticides in countries endemic with or at risk of major vector-borne diseases. *Environmental Health Perspectives*, 2011, 119:1517–1522 (doi:10.1289/ehp.1103637).

[11] van den Berg H et al. Status of pesticide management in the practice of vector control: a global survey in countries at risk of malaria or other major vector-borne diseases. *Malaria Journal*, 2011, 10:125 (doi:10.1186/1475-2875-10-125).

[12] *Guidelines for procuring public health pesticides*. Geneva, World Health Organization, 2012 (WHO/HTM/NTD/WHOPES/2012.4).

[13] *Guidelines for monitoring the durability of long-lasting insecticidal mosquito nets under operational conditions*. Geneva, World Health Organization, 2011 (WHO/HTM/NTD/WHOPES/2011.5).

[14] *Guidelines for testing the efficacy of insecticide products used in aircraft*. Geneva, World Health Organization, 2012 (WHO/HTM/NTD/WHOPES/2012.1).

[15] *Generic risk assessment model for insecticides used for larviciding – first revision.* Geneva, World Health Organization, 2010 (WHO/HTM/NTD/WHOPES/2010.4.Rev1).

[16] *Generic risk assessment model for indoor residual spraying of insecticides — first revision.* Geneva, World Health Organization, 2010 (WHO/HTM/NTD/WHOPES/2010.5.Rev1).

[17] *Generic risk assessment model for indoor and outdoor space spraying of insecticides — first revision.* Geneva, World Health Organization, 2010 (WHO/HTM/NTD/WHOPES/2010.6.Rev1).

[18] http://www.who.int/whopes/recommendations/wgm/en/

4.4   SAFE WATER, SANITATION AND HYGIENE

The WHO/UNICEF Joint Monitoring Programme for Water Supply and Sanitation reports every 2 years on progress made towards achieving the Millennium Development Goal target for drinking-water and sanitation (target 7c: halve, by 2015, the proportion of people without sustainable access to safe drinking-water and basic sanitation). The joint monitoring programme announced in its March 2011 report that the drinking-water target had been reached in 2010, 5 years ahead of the target date, as measured by its proxy indicator: access to and use of improved sources (*1*).

Between 1990 and 2010, more than 2 billion people gained access to improved water sources. The report noted, however, that this leaves some 780 million people in the world without adequate sanitation and safe drinking-water; moreover, the sanitation target remains off-track (2.5 billion: a critical determinant in relation to the burden of many neglected tropical diseases). Moreover, the report showed that there were disparities among different regions of the world (for example, 40% of those without access to improved water sources live in sub-Saharan Africa, where many neglected tropical diseases are prevalent), and that the proxy indicator provides no absolute information about the safety of drinking-water from improved sources.

Although the number of people resorting to open defecation worldwide has decreased by 271 million since 1990, it is still practised by a majority of rural populations in 19 countries, accounting for about 1.1 billion people worldwide or 15% of the population. The biggest challenge is in India, where more than half of the country's population (626 million people) do not have access to basic toilet facilities.

The report also showed that despite 1.8 billion people having gained access to improved sanitation facilities between 1990 and 2010, an estimated 2.5 billion people still live without any improvements to sanitation services, and almost three quarters of them live in rural areas. The world is unlikely to meet the sanitation target by 2015; this will be an impediment to WHO's fight to eliminate some of the 17 neglected tropical diseases.

In January 2012, the outcome of a systematic literature review supported by WHO was published (2) analysing the association between improving sanitation and reducing the risks of transmission for soil-transmitted helminthiases. A positive correlation suggests the value of prioritizing improvements in sanitation together with delivering preventive chemotherapy and health education as a basis for sustaining reductions in the prevalence of helminths.

REFERENCES

[1]   *Progress on drinking water and sanitation: 2012 update.* Geneva, World Health Organization, 2012 (http://www.wssinfo.org/fileadmin/user_upload/resources/JMP-report-2012-en.pdf; accessed December 2012).

[2]   Ziegelbauer K et al. Effect of sanitation on soil-transmitted helminth infection: systematic review and meta-analysis. *PLoS Medicine*, 2012, 9(1):e1001162 (doi:10.1371/journal.pmed.1001162).

4.5   VETERINARY PUBLIC-HEALTH SERVICES TO CONTROL NEGLECTED ZOONOTIC DISEASES

Veterinary public health services consist of understanding and applying veterinary sciences at the human–animal interface to protect human health, particularly against zoonotic diseases and related threats (1). Veterinary public health has been promoted by WHO since its inception (1). In 2008, a new concept, known as "one health", was defined as "the collaborative effort of multiple disciplines to attain optimal health for humans, animals, and our environment" (2). The one-health concept emphasizes detecting and controlling zoonoses by promoting enhanced intersectoral collaboration and communication, ensuring joint planning among relevant ministries, and providing novel cost-effective transsectoral options for controlling zoonoses in low-income countries (3). Veterinary public-health services in ministries of health or agriculture will continue to provide the organizational basis and programme structure to move forward the one-health approach at the national level (4). There is a range of interventions available for preventing and controlling zoonoses (*Fig. 4.5.1*).

KEY INTERVENTIONS: SITUATION REPORT

Fig. 4.5.1 Veterinary public-health interventions[a] available for preventing and controlling neglected zoonotic diseases (NZDs) (*10*)

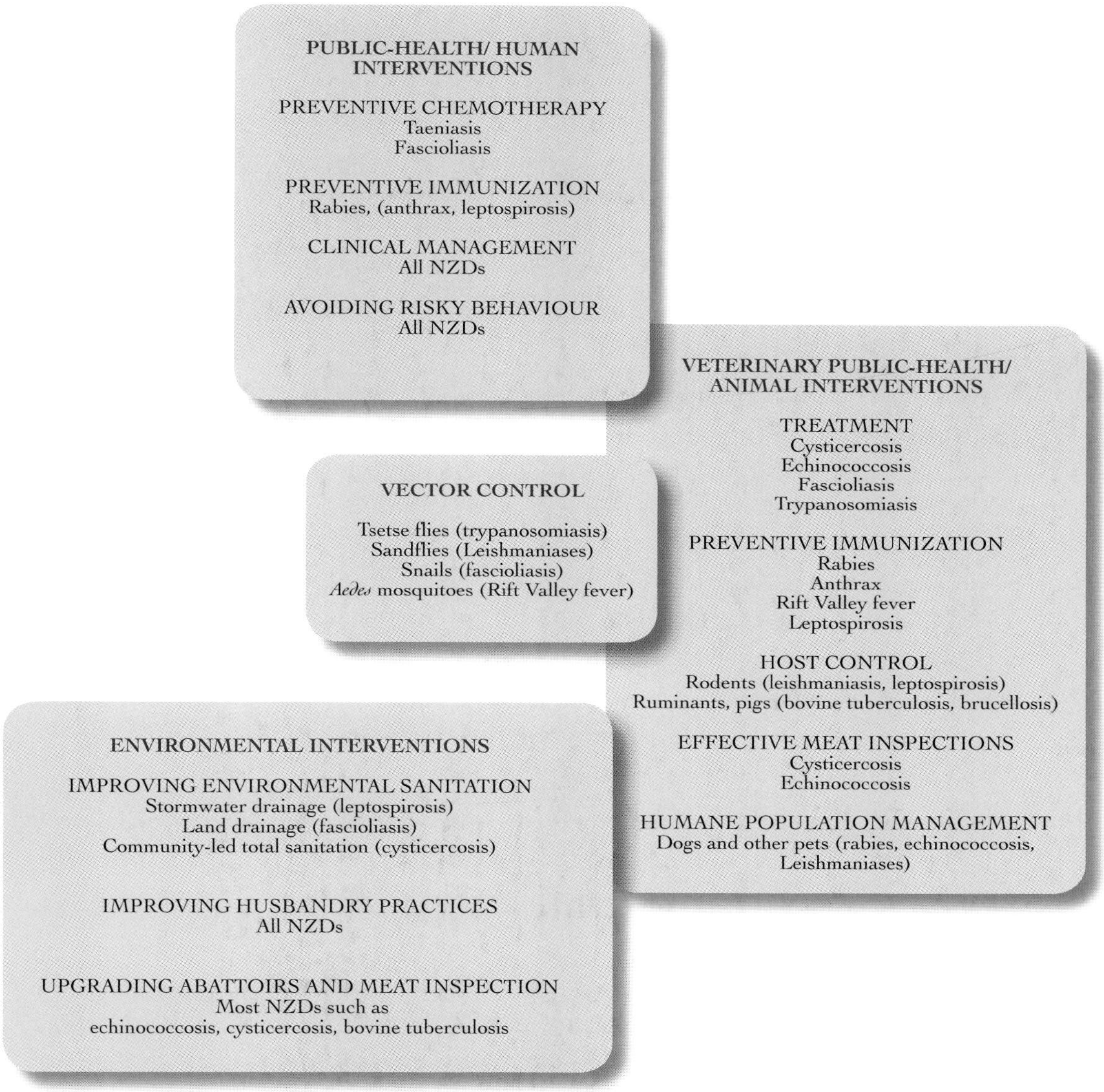

PUBLIC-HEALTH/ HUMAN INTERVENTIONS

PREVENTIVE CHEMOTHERAPY
Taeniasis
Fascioliasis

PREVENTIVE IMMUNIZATION
Rabies, (anthrax, leptospirosis)

CLINICAL MANAGEMENT
All NZDs

AVOIDING RISKY BEHAVIOUR
All NZDs

VECTOR CONTROL

Tsetse flies (trypanosomiasis)
Sandflies (Leishmaniases)
Snails (fascioliasis)
Aedes mosquitoes (Rift Valley fever)

VETERINARY PUBLIC-HEALTH/ ANIMAL INTERVENTIONS

TREATMENT
Cysticercosis
Echinococcosis
Fascioliasis
Trypanosomiasis

PREVENTIVE IMMUNIZATION
Rabies
Anthrax
Rift Valley fever
Leptospirosis

HOST CONTROL
Rodents (leishmaniasis, leptospirosis)
Ruminants, pigs (bovine tuberculosis, brucellosis)

EFFECTIVE MEAT INSPECTIONS
Cysticercosis
Echinococcosis

HUMANE POPULATION MANAGEMENT
Dogs and other pets (rabies, echinococcosis, Leishmaniases)

ENVIRONMENTAL INTERVENTIONS

IMPROVING ENVIRONMENTAL SANITATION
Stormwater drainage (leptospirosis)
Land drainage (fascioliasis)
Community-led total sanitation (cysticercosis)

IMPROVING HUSBANDRY PRACTICES
All NZDs

UPGRADING ABATTOIRS AND MEAT INSPECTION
Most NZDs such as
echinococcosis, cysticercosis, bovine tuberculosis

[a] All interventions need to be mobilized for effective control of zoonoses, including preventive chemotherapy, preventive immunization and clinical management of human disease, vector control, and those taking place in the environment and at the human–animal interface.

As in the case of NTDs, there are a number of human diseases that are transmitted from animals (zoonoses) that have tended to be forgotten or overlooked (*5*). These zoonoses are best defined by the people and communities they most affect: poor people living in remote rural areas or urban slums in the developing world (*6,7*). They have been named neglected zoonotic diseases to indicate that they have been insufficiently addressed by governments and the international community as interest has shifted to newly emerging zoonoses, particularly those with the potential for pandemic spread. The term neglected zoonotic diseases is accepted internationally (*8–10*). These endemic zoonoses negatively affect the health and productivity of livestock, causing infertility, death, low yields of milk, and by rendering meat inedible (*11*). Thus, they impose a burden on the health of both humans and animals in the populations least able to cope with such problems (*8–10*).

Examples of neglected zoonotic diseases are cysticercosis and taeniasis caused by infection with *Taenia solium*, cystic echinococcosis, human rabies transmitted by dogs, and zoonotic human African trypanosomiasis (*8–10*). As international awareness of these diseases has increased, and a clearer idea of their characteristics has emerged, the list of neglected zoonoses has continued to grow. The neglected zoonotic diseases that are included in the list of 17 NTDs are cystic echinococcosis, fascioliasis and other *T. solium* foodborne trematodiases, human rabies transmitted by dogs, cysticercosis, zoonotic trypanosomiasis and the Leishmaniases (*5*).

The third international conference on neglected zoonotic diseases was held at WHO's Geneva headquarters in November 2010. The conference identified five points for urgent attention (*10*):

- ensuring that assessments of the burden of zoonoses take into account their dual burden on the health of humans and of livestock, and thus their total cost to society;

- prioritizing studies on multidisease packages and host approaches for selected neglected zoonotic diseases in order to improve and sustain the cost effectiveness of efforts to control these diseases;

- scaling up interventions for control and elimination when feasible in selected geographical and epidemiological settings;

- promoting collaboration among sectors such as health, livestock, agriculture, natural resources and wildlife, and developing policies across sectors;

- strengthening advocacy for control of these diseases among stakeholders by informing them about the societal burden of these diseases, and providing education to affected populations to create demand for control at all levels of society.

A proposal for investment in veterinary public-health services for a prioritized portfolio of neglected zoonotic diseases was developed at an interagency meeting (*12*). The portfolio comprises:

- three neglected diseases of global importance (*T. solium* cysticercosis and taeniasis, cystic echinococcosis and rabies transmitted to humans by dogs); plus

KEY INTERVENTIONS: SITUATION REPORT

- two neglected diseases of regional importance (fascioliasis and other foodborne trematodiases, and zoonotic trypanosomiasis); plus
- control activities focusing on major bacterial zoonoses (anthrax, brucellosis and leptospirosis).

The first evaluation of costs indicated that a minimum of US $20 million per year in external funding is needed for 5 years (2012–2016) to achieve the expected outcomes by 2016.

Provided that political commitment and adequate resources are available then rabies, a leading viral neglected zoonotic disease, should be eliminated from the Region of the Americas by 2015, and from the South-East Asia Region by 2020. Activities to accelerate control of parasitic neglected zoonotic diseases must take place during the next 8 years (*15*).

REFERENCES

[1] *Future trends in veterinary public health: report of a WHO study group.* Geneva, World Health Organization, 2002 (WHO Technical Report Series, No. 907).

[2] *One Health: a new professional initiative.* Schaumburg, IL, American Veterinary Medical Association, 2008 (https://www.avma.org/KB/Resources/Reports/Documents/onehealth_final.pdf; accessed September 2012).

[3] Zinsstag J, Tanner M. "One health": the potential of closer cooperation between human and animal health in Africa, *Swiss Tropical Institute*, Basel, Switzerland. http://www.swisstph.ch/datensatzsammlung/newsletter/newslettermarch08/onehealthzinsstag.htm

[4] Arambulo P. Veterinary public health in the age of "one health". *Journal of the American Veterinary Medical Association*, 2011, 239:48–49.

[5] *Working to overcome the global impact of neglected tropical diseases: first WHO report on neglected tropical diseases.* Geneva, World Health Organization, 2010 (WHO/HTM/NTD/2010.1).

[6] Doble L, Fèvre EM. Focusing on neglected zoonoses. *The Veterinary Record*, 2010, 166: 546–547.

[7] Molyneux D et al. Zoonoses and marginalised infectious diseases of poverty: where do we stand? *Parasites and Vectors*, 2011, 4:1–19.

[8] *The control of neglected zoonotic diseases: a route to poverty alleviation.* Geneva, World Health Organization, 2006 (WHO/SDE/FOS/2006.1).

[9] *Integrated control of neglected zoonotic diseases in Africa: applying the "One Health" concept.* Geneva, World Health Organization, 2008 (WHO/HTM/NTD/NZD/2008.1).

[10] *The control of neglected zoonotic diseases: community-based interventions for prevention and control.* Geneva, World Health Organization, 2011 (WHO/HTM/NTD/NZD/2011.1).

[11] Randolph TF et al. Role of livestock in human nutrition and health for poverty reduction in developing countries. *Journal of Animal Science*, 2007, 85:2788–2800.

[12] *Interagency meeting on planning the prevention and control of neglected zoonotic diseases (NZDs).* Geneva, World Health Organization, 2011 (WHO/HTM/NTD/NZD/2011.3).

[13] *Accelerating work to overcome the global impact of neglected tropical diseases: a roadmap for implementation.* Geneva, World Health Organization, 2012 (WHO/HTM/NTD 2012.1).

4.6   CAPACITY STRENGTHENING

One of WHO's key capacity-strengthening activities is providing the conditions that allow all health-care staff to develop the skills necessary to manage efficiently national control programmes that target neglected tropical diseases. WHO is responsible for formulating appropriate training and for strengthening implementation capacity so that programmes can respond more effectively and deliver integrated control strategies (*1*).

As donations of medicines increased, and interventions were scaled up, WHO convened a Working Group on Capacity Strengthening. The working group's mandate is to strengthen country-level capacity by ensuring that managers of national programmes and and health-care providers are well trained so that control programmes targeting NTDs will be sustained.

Consistent with WHO's global plan to combat NTDs (*2*), and based on guidance provided by the Strategic and Technical Advisory Group for Neglected Tropical Diseases, the working group has prioritized the need to strengthen country-level capacity (with assistance from donors and support from regional offices) by:

- identifying existing capacity-strengthening efforts;

- recognizing gaps in efforts, and prioritizing capacity-strengthening needs that must be addressed in both the short term and the long term;

- advising, standardizing and supporting the implementation of training curricula to strengthen managerial and technical capacity for NTD control;

- harmonizing partners' efforts to increase their contributions to ensure that identifiable needs are met.

An international training workshop for managers of national programmes was organized by WHO in collaboration with the United States Agency for International

Development's NTD Program and its new flagship project "Envision". The training session was piloted in Pemba, United Republic of Tanzania, at the WHO collaborating centre in July 2012. The aim of the training was to develop the capacity of national NTD programme managers to manage preventive chemotherapy control programmes in compliance with WHO's standards and guidelines. Training activities will be increased during 2013 and 2014. During this time, WHO will also look at strengthening capacity:

- for controlling diseases that require intensified disease-management, and for which specific clinical, treatment and surveillance skills are needed;

- by training personnel to support a coordinated scaling up of effective vector-control programmes in areas where human resources in medical entomology have declined;

- in order to enhance integrated approaches to human health and animal health.

REFERENCES

[1] *Accelerating work to overcome the global impact of neglected tropical diseases: a roadmap for implementation.* Geneva, World Health Organization, 2012 (WHO/HTM/NTD/2012.1).

[2] *Global plan to combat neglected tropical diseases 2008–2015.* Geneva, World Health Organization, 2007 (WHO/CDS/NTD/2007.3).

ANNEXES

ANNEXES

Annex 1. Resolutions of the World Health Assembly (WHA) concerning neglected tropical diseases, 1948–2012

Disease	WHA resolution number	Title	Year
Vector-borne disease	WHA1.12	Vector biology and control	1948
Vector-borne disease	WHA2.18	Expert Committee on insecticides: report on the first session	1949
Endemic treponematoses	WHA2.36	Bejel and other treponematoses	1949
Leprosy	WHA2.43	Leprosy	1949
Rabies	WHA3.20	Rabies	1950
Trachoma	WHA3.22	Trachoma	1950
Hydatidosis	WHA3.23	Hydatidosis	1950
Schistosomiasis and soil-transmitted helminthiases	WHA3.26	Bilharziasis	1950
Vector-borne disease	WHA3.43	Labelling and distribution of insecticides	1950
Trachoma	WHA4.29	Trachoma	1951
Vector-borne disease	WHA4.30	Supply of insecticides	1951
Leprosy	WHA5.28	Leprosy	1952
Vector-borne disease	WHA5.29	Supply and requirements of insecticides: world position	1952
Leprosy	WHA6.19	Expert Committee on leprosy: first report	1953
Leprosy	WHA9.45	Inter-regional conference on leprosy control, 1958	1956
Vector-borne disease	WHA13.54	Vector-borne diseases and malaria eradication	1960
Vector-borne disease	WHA22.40	Research on methods of vector control	1969
Vector-borne disease	WHA23.33	Research on alternative methods of vector control	1970
Research	WHA27.52	Intensification of research on tropical parasitic diseases	1974
Leprosy	WHA27.58	Coordination and strengthening of leprosy control	1974
Schistosomiasis	WHA28.53	Schistosomiasis	1975
Avoidable blindness (for both onchocerciasis and trachoma)	WHA28.54	Prevention of blindness	1975
Leprosy	WHA28.56	Leprosy control	1975
Research	WHA28.71	WHO's role in the development and coordination of research in tropical diseases	1975
Schistosomiasis	WHA29.58	Schistosomiasis	1976
Leprosy	WHA29.70	Leprosy control	1976
Leprosy	WHA30.36	Leprosy control	1977
Research	WHA30.42	Special Programme for Research and Training in Tropical Diseases	1977
Zoonoses	WHA31.48	Prevention and control of zoonoses and foodborne diseases due to animal products	1978
Endemic treponematoses	WHA31.58	Control of endemic treponematoses	1978
Leprosy	WHA32.39	Leprosy	1979
Dracunculiasis	WHA34.25	International drinking-water supply and sanitation decade	1981
Human African trypanosomiasis	WHA36.31	African human trypanosomiasis	1983
Dracunculiasis	WHA39.21	Elimination of dracunculiasis	1986
Leprosy	WHA40.35	Towards the elimination of leprosy	1987

Annex 1. (continued)

Disease	WHA resolution number	Title	Year
Dracunculiasis	WHA42.25	International Drinking Water Supply and Sanitation Decade	1989
Dracunculiasis	WHA42.29	Elimination of dracunculiasis	1989
Vector-borne disease	WHA42.31	Control of disease vectors and pests	1989
Research	WHA43.18	Tropical disease research	1990
Dracunculiasis	WHA44.5	Eradication of dracunculiasis	1991
Leprosy	WHA44.9	Leprosy	1991
Dengue and dengue haemorrhagic fever	WHA46.31	Dengue prevention and control	1993
Onchocerciasis	WHA47.32	Onchocerciasis control through ivermectin distribution	1994
Vector-borne disease	WHA50.13	Promotion of chemical safety, with special attention to persistent organic pollutants	1997
Lymphatic filariasis	WHA50.29	Elimination of lymphatic filariasis as a public health problem	1997
Dracunculiasis	WHA50.35	Eradication of dracunculiasis	1997
Human African trypanosomiasis	WHA50.36	African trypanosomiasis	1997
Trachoma	WHA51.11	Global elimination of blinding trachoma	1998
Chagas disease	WHA51.14	Elimination of transmission of Chagas disease	1998
Leprosy	WHA51.15	Elimination of leprosy as a public health problem	1998
Schistosomiasis and soil-transmitted helminthiases	WHA54.19	Schistosomiasis and soil-transmitted helminth Infections	2001
Dengue and dengue haemorrhagic fever	WHA55.17	Prevention and control of dengue fever and dengue haemorrhagic fever	2002
Human African trypanosomiasis	WHA56.7	Pan African tsetse and trypanosomiasis eradication campaign	2003
Avoidable blindness (for both onchocerciasis and trachoma)	WHA56.26	Elimination of avoidable blindness	2003
Buruli ulcer	WHA57.1	Surveillance and control of Mycobacterium ulcerans disease (Buruli ulcer)	2004
Human African trypanosomiasis	WHA57.2	Control of human African trypanosomiasis	2004
Dracunculiasis	WHA57.9	Eradication of dracunculiasis	2004
Avoidable blindness (for both onchocerciasis and trachoma)	WHA59.25	Prevention of avoidable blindness and visual impairment	2006
Leishmaniases	WHA60.13	Control of leishmaniasis	2007
Avoidable blindness (for both onchocerciasis and trachoma)	WHA62.1	Prevention of avoidable blindness and visual impairment	2009
Chagas disease	WHA63.20	Chagas disease: control and elimination	2010
Vector-borne disease	WHA63.26	Improvement of health through sound management of obsolete pesticides and other obsolete chemicals	2010
Dracunculiasis	WHA64.16	Eradication of dracunculiasis	2011
Schistosomiasis	WHA65.21	Elimination of schistosomiasis	2012

Annex 2. Medicines for controlling neglected tropical diseases donated by the pharmaceutical industry

Pharmaceutical company	Medicine	Donation
Bayer	Nifurtimox	Up to 400 000 tablets per year during 2009-2014 for human African trypanosomiasis; donation made through WHO
	Nifurtimox	Up to 1 million tablets per year during 2012-2017 for second-line treatment of Chagas disease; donation made through WHO
	Suramin	Up to 10 000 vials per year until November 2012 for human African trypanosomiasis; donation made through WHO
Eisai	Diethylcarbamazine	Up to 2.2 billion tablets until 2020 for lymphatic filariasis; donation made through WHO
Gilead Sciences	AmBisome	Up to 445 000 vials during 2012–2017 for visceral leishmaniasis in South-East Asia and East Africa; donation made through WHO
GlaxoSmithKline	Albendazole	Unlimited supply for as long as needed for lymphatic filariasis and soil-transmitted helminthiases; donation made through WHO
Johnson & Johnson	Mebendazole	Up to 200 million tablets per year until 2020 for soil-transmitted helminthiases control programmes for school-age children; donation made through WHO
Merck & Co., Inc.,	Ivermectin	Unlimited supply for as long as needed; donation made directly to countries for lymphatic filariasis and onchocerciasis
Merck KGaA	Praziquantel	Up to 250 million tablets per year for unlimited period for schistosomiasis; donation made through WHO
Novartis	Multidrug therapy (rifampicin, clofazimine and dapsone in blister packs) and loose tablets of clofazimine	Unlimited supply for as long as needed for leprosy and its complications; donation made through WHO
	Triclabendazole	Up to 600 000 tablets annually for fascioliasis and paragonimiasis; donation made through WHO
Pfizer	Azithromycin	Unlimited quantity for blinding trachoma until at least 2020
Sanofi	Eflornithine	Unlimited quantity until 2020 for human African trypanosomiasis; donation made through WHO
	Melarsoprol	Unlimited quantity until 2020 for human African trypanosomiasis; donation made through WHO
	Pentamidine	Unlimited quantity until 2020 for human African trypanosomiasis; donation made through WHO
	Notezine (Diethylcarbamazine)	120 million tablets with support from Eisai and the Bill & Melinda Gates Foundation for 2012–2013; donation made through WHO

Annex 3a. Targets and milestones for eliminating[1] and eradicating[2] neglected tropical diseases, 2015–2020

DISEASE	2015				2020			
	Eradication	Global elimination	Regional elimination	Country elimination	Eradication	Global elimination	Regional elimination	Country elimination
Rabies[b]			√ Latin America				√ South-East Asia and Western Pacific regions	
Blinding trachoma						√		
Endemic treponematoses (yaws)					√			
Leprosy						√		
Chagas disease			√ Transmission through blood transfusion interrupted				√ Intra-domiciliary transmission interrupted in the Region of the Americas	
Human African trypanosomiasis				√ In 80% of foci		√		
Visceral leishmaniasis							√ Indian subcontinent	
Dracunculiasis	√							
Lymphatic filariasis						√		
Onchocerciasis			√ Latin America	√ Yemen				√ Selected countries in Africa
Schistosomiasis			√ Eastern Mediterranean Region, Caribbean, Indonesia and the Mekong River basin				√ Region of the Americas and Western Pacific Region	√ Selected countries in Africa

[1] Elimination (interruption of transmission) is the reduction to zero of the incidence of infection caused by a specific pathogen in a defined geographical area as a result of deliberate efforts; continued actions to prevent re-establishment of transmission may be required (see Section 2.1).

[2] Eradication is the permanent reduction to zero of the worldwide incidence of infection caused by a specific pathogen as a result of deliberate efforts, with no risk of reintroduction. In some cases a pathogen may become extinct, but others may be present in confined settings, such as laboratories (see Section 2.1).

Annex 3b. Targets and milestones for intensifying control[1] of neglected tropical diseases, 2015–2020

DISEASE	2015	2020
Dengue	• Sustainable dengue vector control interventions established in10 endemic priority countries	• Dengue control and surveillance systems established in all regions • Number of cases reduced by more than 25% (2009–2010 as base line) and deaths by 50%
Buruli ulcer	• Study completed and oral antibiotic therapy incorporated into control and treatment	• 70% of all cases detected early and cured with antibiotics in all endemic countries
Cutaneous leishmaniasis	• 70% of all cases detected and at least 90% of all detected cases treated in the Eastern Mediterranean Region	
Taeniasis/cysticercosis and echinococcosis	• Validated strategy for control and elimination of *T. solium* taeniasis/cysticercosis available • Pilot projects to validate effective echinococcosis control strategies implemented in selected countries as a public-health problem	• Interventions scaled up in selected countries for *T. solium* taeniasis/cysticercosis control and elimination • Validated strategy available for echinococcosis and interventions scaled up in selected countries for their control and elimination
Foodborne trematode infections	• Foodborne trematode infections included in mainstream preventive chemotherapy strategy • • Morbidity due to foodborne trematode infections controlled where feasible	• 75% of population at risk reached by preventive chemotherapy Morbidity due to foodborne trematode infections controlled in all endemic countries
Soil-transmitted helminthiases (intestinal worms)	• 50% of preschool and school-aged children in need of treatment are regularly treated • 100% of countries have a plan of action	• 75% of preschool and school-aged children in need of treatment are regularly treated • 75% coverage achieved in preschool and school-aged children in 100% of countries

[1] Control is the reduction of disease incidence, prevalence, intensity, morbidity, or mortality, or a combination of these, as a result of deliberate efforts. The term "elimination as a public-health problem" should be used only upon achievement of measurable targets for control set by Member States in relation to a specific disease. Continued intervention measures may be required to maintain this reduction.

ANNEXES

Annex 4. Operational definitions and indicators for eradication targets and elimination targets as defined in the roadmap for implementation (*Annex 3a*)

Target	Disease/Condition	Scope	Operational definition	Indicator(s)
ERADICATION				
	Dracunculiasis	(WHA 64.16, 2011) (Guinea worm disease)	Interruption of transmission of *Dracunculus medinensis* (leading to zero incidence of indigenous guinea-worm disease cases for at least one year after last indigenous case). Certified after a minimum period of three consecutive years of adequate surveillance.[1]	Incidence of indigenous cases
	Endemic treponematoses	(WHA 31.58, 1978)	Interruption of transmission of *Treponema pallidum pertenue*, *T. p. endemicum* and *Treponema carateum* (zero incidence of yaws, bejel and pinta). Certification criteria to be defined.	Incidence of cases
ELIMINATION				
	Blinding Trachoma	Global elimination as a public health problem (WHA51.11, 1998)	Incidence of less than one case of blindness due to trachoma per 1000 population in each endemic country. Verified after a minimum period of three consecutive years of adequate post-intervention surveillance.	Prevalence of unmanaged trachomatous trichiasis in all ages; prevalence of trachoma follicular in children 1 to 9 years coverage of FE interventions.[2]
	Chagas disease	Regional elimination (WHA63.20, 2010)	Interruption of transmission of *Trypanosoma cruzi* through blood transfusion and intra-domiciliary vectors.	Incidence of cases transmitted by intra-domiciliary vectors; Coverage of blood banks implementing preventive screening policies
	Human African trypanosomiasis	Global elimination as a public health problem (WHA 57.2, 2004)	Very low prevalence of disease due to *Trypanosma brucei gambiense* and *T. b. rhodesiense* in all endemic foci. Criteria to be defined by WHO group of experts.	Number of new cases
	Leprosy	Global elimination as a public health problem (WHA 51.15, 1998)	Reduction of new cases with Grade 2 disabilities due to *Mycobacterium leprae* below one per million population.	Incidence of cases with Grade 2 disabilities
	Lymphatic filariasis	Global elimination as a public health problem (WHA 50.29, 1997)	Prevalence of infection with *Wuchereria bancrofti*, *Brugia malayi* or *B. timori* less than target thresholds in all endemic areas in all countries.	Prevalence as defined for the various species/vector complexes in Transmission Assessment Surveys (TAS).[3]
	Onchocerciasis	Regional and country elimination (CD48.R12, 2008)	Prevalence of infection with *Onchocerca volvulus* less than target threshold in children less than 10 years old, and prevalence of infective larvae in *Simulium* flies less than target threshold. Verified after a minimum period of 3-5 consecutive years of adequate post-intervention surveillance.	Prevalence of specific antibodies in children and prevalence of infective larvae in *Simulium* flies.[4]
	Rabies	Regional elimination (WHA3.20, 1950)	Interruption of dog to dog rabies transmission with absence of human rabies cases due to a dog virus for 2 consecutive years.	Incidence of animal and human rabies transmitted by dogs.
		Elimination: sub-regional (Caribbean); country (Indonesia, selected countries in Eastern Mediterranean) (WHA65.21, 2012)	Reduction of incidence of infection with any of the human *Schistosoma* species to zero.	Incidence of cases in children born after reported interruption of transmission; presence of parasite-specific DNA detected in intermediate snail hosts.[5]
	Visceral leishmaniasis	Regional elimination as public health problem in SEAR (WHA60.13)	Incidence of visceral leishmaniasis below one case per 10 000 population per year at district and sub-district levels.	Incidence of cases

[1] WHO, 1996. *Certification of dracunculiasis eradication. Criteria, strategies, procedures.* WHO/FIL/96.188 Rev.1.

[2] WHO, 2006. *Trachoma control: a guide for programme managers.* ISBN 92 4 154690 5

[3] WHO, 2011. *Monitoring and epidemiological assessment of mass drug administration in the global programme to eliminate lymphatic filariasis: a manual for national elimination programmes.* WHO/HTM/NTD/PCT/2011; ISBN 978 92 4 150148 4.

[4] WHO, in press. *Assessment of elimination of human onchocerciasis: criteria and procedures.* Revised version.

[5] WHO, 2013. *Schistosomiasis: progress report 2001–2011 and strategic plan 2012–2020.*

[6] Criteria and guidelines under development, as requested by WHA 65.21.

Annex 5. Methods used to prepare maps and charts

Population

The total population of each country is taken from *World population prospects: 2010 revision* (*1*). In some cases, the population of children aged 1–4 years and 5–14 years is also given since these are the age groups specifically targeted for anthelminthic treatments.

Preventive chemotherapy data

Unless otherwise specified, data on preventive chemotherapy are as provided by national authorities to WHO through reporting processes in country and regional offices using standardized templates. Maps and charts for lymphatic filariasis, soil-transmitted helminthiases, schistosomiasis, onchocerciasis and trachoma were prepared using data reported to WHO annually. Information from the Preventive Chemotherapy and Transmission Control Databank was used to compile sections of this report, and is accessible online (*2*).

The main definitions of data used to describe preventive chemotherapy are as follows:

- **population requiring preventive chemotherapy** – the total population living in all endemic areas that requires preventive chemotherapy;

- **geographical coverage** – the proportion (%) of endemic districts covered by preventive chemotherapy;

- **programme coverage** – the proportion (%) of individuals who were treated according to the programme's target;

- **national disease-specific coverage** – the proportion (%) of individuals in the population requiring preventive chemotherapy for the specific disease that was treated.

Dracunculiasis data are reported weekly to WHO by national authorities that provide updates on the status of the eradication initiative at the country level as well as related epidemiological information.

Fascioliasis data are based on information obtained from peer-reviewed publications, and supplemented by the opinions of international experts.

Data on innovative and intensified disease-management

Data for neglected tropical diseases in which the large-scale use of existing tools is limited have been obtained by various non-integrated methods that depend on the particulars of the disease-control programme. Details of the data sources are given below:

- **Chagas disease** – data reported to WHO as official estimates and endorsed through a consultative process among national authorities and international experts;

- **Buruli ulcer** – annual data reported to WHO by national authorities using a standardized template;

- **Endemic syphilis** – historical data and ad hoc information reported to WHO by national authorities and researchers;

- **Human African trypanosomiasis** – data reported to WHO annually by national authorities using a standardized template;

- **Leishmaniases** – ad hoc information made available to WHO by programme managers and researchers;

- **Leprosy** – data reported to WHO annually by national authorities using a standardized template.

Zoonoses data

- **Rabies** – Data are based on information obtained from peer-reviewed publications, and supplemented by the opinions of international experts.

- **Cysticercosis** – Data are based on information obtained from peer-reviewed publications, and supplemented by the opinions of international experts.

- **Echinococcosis** – Data are based on information obtained from peer-reviewed publications, and the opinions of international experts.

Annex 5. (continued)

Sources of information for figures and chapters

Sources of information are mostly indicated in each figure and specific chapter. All reasonable precautions have been taken to verify and confirm the accuracy of the information contained in this publication.

REFERENCES

[1] *World population prospects: 2010 revision.* New York, NY, United Nations Population Division, 2010 (http://esa.un.org/wpp/index.htm).

[2] *Preventive chemotherapy and transmission control databank.* Geneva, World Health Organization, 2010 (http://www.who.int/neglected_diseases/preventive_chemotherapy/databank/en/; accessed December 2012).

WHO REGIONAL OFFICES

Regional Office for Africa
Cité du Djoué, P.O.Box 06
Brazzaville, Congo
Telephone: + 242 839 100 / +47 241 39100
Facsimile: + 242 839 501 / +47 241 395018
E-mail: regafro@afro.who.int

Regional Office for the Americas
525, 23rd Street, N.W.
Washington, DC 20037, USA
Telephone: +1 202 974 3000
Facsimile: +1 202 974 3663
E-mail: postmaster@paho.org

Regional Office for South-East Asia
World Health House
Indraprastha Estate
Mahatama Gandhi Marg
New Delhi 110 002, India
Telephone: + 91-11-2337 0804
Facsimile: + 91-11-2337 9507
E-mail: guptasmithv@searo.who.int

Regional Office for Europe
8, Scherfigsvej
DK-2100 Copenhagen 0, Denmark
Telephone: + 45 39 171 717
Facsimile: + 45 39 171 818
E-mail: postmaster@euro.who.int

Regional Office for the Eastern Mediterranean
Abdul Razzak Al Sanhouri Street
P.O. Box 7608
Nasr City, Cairo 11371, Egypt
Telephone: + 202 2276 50 00
Facsimile: + 202 2670 24 92 or 2670 24 94
E-mail: postmaster@emro.who.int

Regional Office for the Western Pacific
P.O. Box 2932
1000 Manila, Philippines
Telephone: + 63 2 528 8001
E-mail: postmaster@wpro.who.int